Working Alongside People with Long Term Mental Health Problems

Working Alongside People with Long Term Mental Health Problems

Rachel Perkins
Pathfinder Mental Health Services Trust
London
UK

and

Julie Repper
Sheffield Centre for Health and Related Research
Sheffield
UK

Stanley Thornes (Publishers) Ltd

First published in 1996 by Chapman & Hall

Reprinted in 1999 by:
Stanley Thornes (Publishers) Ltd
Ellenborough House
Wellington Street
Cheltenham
Glos.
GL50 1YW
United Kingdom

99 00 01 02 03 / 10 9 8 7 6 5 4 3 2 1

A catalogue record for this book is available from the British Library

ISBN 0–7487–5171–8

Typeset by Saxon Graphics Ltd, Derby
Printed and bound in Great Britain by Athenaeum Press Ltd, Gateshead, Tyne & Wear

Contents

Introduction

Over recent years, services for people who are disabled by serious ongoing mental health problems have been accorded increased priority and attention. For many working in the mental health field, this has required a marked departure from the practice in which they have hitherto been engaged: work with those whose mental distress is less severe. For those already focusing on more disabled people, the development of care in the community has wrought great changes in the services in which they work, and the rising user movements have significantly altered the values underpinning their day to day practice. Whilst people severely disabled by mental health problems once spent the majority of their lives in the back wards of large remote mental hospitals, now all moves are to enable such people to live as ordinary a life as possible within the communities of which they are a part.

It is within this context that we have written this book. It is a text for anyone who is already working with those who experience serious and ongoing mental health problems, or who is entering such work, or who simply wishes to extend their understanding and skills. It is intended for all professionals and non-professionals working within health and social services and in independent or voluntary sectors. Psychiatrists, nurses, social workers, psychologists, occupational therapists, physiotherapists, arts therapists, welfare rights workers, legal advisers and volunteers all bring a unique expertise and contribution, but there are many general considerations and approaches that are of relevance to everyone working in the field. It is towards these that the present text is directed. It aims to enable people from all disciplines and areas of expertise to consider the goals and underpinning assumptions and philosophies of their work and to use the skills that they already possess to maximum effect in the service of those who are disabled by serious mental health problems.

Services for people who experience serious long term mental health problems have been the subject of numerous good texts (for example, Wing and Morris, 1981; Shepherd, 1984; Lavender and Holloway, 1988; Ekdawi and Conning, 1994) which outline the philosophies underpinning service development together with the range of supports, interventions and facilities necessary to provide effective care. It is not our intention to replicate this work in the present volume. In our clinical work, teaching and training we have become increasingly aware of the relative absence of texts which seek to guide work with individual clients. Ordinary experience rarely equips us with an understanding of how to relate to, and form relationships with, people who have major disabilities of cognition and emotion. Someone whose behaviour appears unpredictable and incomprehensible and who describes unusual experiences often engenders feelings of fear – a sense of being unable to cope – in a non-disabled person who does not share their reality. Just how do we interact with someone who believes themselves to be the son of the Queen, who believes that everyone is plotting against them, who believes that a rat has entered her brain and is looking out of her eyes? Most professional training offers little guidance in this regard other than dismissive axioms like 'never collude with a delusion'. The training of most professions is focused on problem removal: presumes that most people will need help for only short periods after which they will be able to function unaided. When faced with someone whose mental health problems are ongoing – someone who is socially disabled – many people feel deskilled.

In this book we have addressed the basic issues of how non-disabled people can come to understand, relate to and effectively help people who have serious ongoing mental health problems. The issues we raise cut across service settings and structures: they are applicable whether one is working in a residential, day or outreach service.

At the outset we must emphasize that this is no 'cookery book': there is no set recipe for working with people whose life, perceptions and experiences we do not share. In all situations, a person's behaviour is determined by the way in which they understand or construe their situation. This applies to mental health workers and disabled clients alike. Throughout this text we have, therefore, focused on different ways of understanding the experiences of a person with serious mental health problems. We then consider the implications of these for relationship formation, intervention and support, but we would urge the reader to refrain from using the examples we give as a prescriptive 'how to' guide. Forming effective relationships and supporting people who have serious mental health problems is a skilled art that must be tailored to each individual and their own unique circumstances. Creativity and ingenuity are as essential as a sensitive understanding of the person's wants, wishes and feelings. In this text we offer an approach to understanding and exploring an individual's world and a variety of ideas drawn from our own experience and that of people disabled by mental health problems whom we have had the privilege to know. It is these people who have acted as our most influential teachers and guides, and many have seen and commented on sections of the text. We are enormously grateful for the time and perseverance they have shown in helping us to gain a glimpse of the rich fabric of their lives.

Both of us have been committed to working with those who have serious mental health problems for our entire careers. Between us we have more than 30 years experience of work in this area. In a field where 'burn out' is so frequently reported, our interest and enthusiasm has grown over this time: fuelled by a liking of, and respect for, those people whom we serve and a firmly held belief that they have an important contribution to make to the lives of our communities. This commitment is not simply driven by a professional interest, we both believe passionately that people who have serious mental health problems have a right to full citizenship and to be a part of the communities in which we live. We have pursued this belief at both a professional and political level, within our work and outside, and will continue to do so. But this is not an act of altruism. The communities in which all of us live are made poorer places when deprived of the contribution of those who have been marginalized and excluded as a consequence of their mental health problems. Even in an era of 'community care', segregation still exists in specialist accommodation, work and day facilities: real integration and involvement is a rarity for many who are seriously disabled by ongoing mental health problems.

We met each other over a decade ago working in a rehabilitation and continuing care service in south London: Julie as a nurse, Rachel as a clinical psychologist. Since this time we have worked together in a variety of clinical, research and teaching capacities. The ideas we present are the product of 15 years of joint and separate work, shared argument and debate. After leaving clinical practice to work as a lecturer in nursing studies, Julie is now a Research Fellow in a health service research unit. Rachel began her career as a lecturer and clinician specializing in work with people with serious ongoing mental health problems and is now a consultant clinical psychologist and Clinical Director of a rehabilitation and continuing community care service in London. Both separately and together we have been involved in several research projects in the area of rehabilitation and continuing community care. We have written widely in the area, frequently present papers at national and international conferences, and regularly provide training for mental health workers from all disciplines working in a range of agencies. However, our understanding of mental health problems does not come from our work alone: we have had first-hand experience of Rachel's own mental health problems. With a diagnosis of manic depressive illness, the writing of this book was punctuated by admission to a psychiatric hospital.

The ideas we present will be considered by some to be controversial. We would ask the reader not to dismiss them out of hand, but to think about them and consider their implications. We start from the belief that people with serious ongoing mental health problems have a right of access to roles, relationships, activities and facilities in the communities of their choice: to move beyond a physical presence in communities to genuinely becoming a part of them. Within this framework, the main role of services is to facilitate and support such access – to enable people to lead the lives they wish. All supports and interventions should be directed towards this end, whether they be pharmacological, psychological or social. We need to move away from a perspective that considers 'patients in our services' to a notion of being there to serve people: to enable them to do the things they want to do by providing help and support that is acceptable to them.

Ensuring access does not, however, mean solely, or even primarily, changing the individual so that they can 'fit in'. If access is to become a reality then at least as much effort must be placed on changing communities so that they can accommodate the disabled individual. Neither does access apply solely to opportunities outside the health care system, it applies equally to mental and physical health services themselves. In this context, access relates not simply to the provision of aids, and help to get to and engage in services, but also to making services attractive and acceptable to the people who need them. We need to move towards providing people with what they want. Most mental health services operate on the explicit or implicit assumption that serious mental health problems prevent a person from accurately judging what they need, therefore staff must make decisions for them, in their own interests, of course. This inaccurate and arrogant assumption has driven many people who need help away from service contact. As with other service industries, we need to adopt the principle that the customer is right. In our experience, even the most disabled people can tell us what they want – it may require time and a will to understand, but it is possible. The main barrier to people telling us what they want is our failure to hear, and act on, what they are saying.

It is never possible for a non-disabled person to fully understand what life looks like from the perspective of one who is disabled: those for whom we provide services are the experts in this regard. However, we can recognize and benefit from this expertise and tailor the assistance we provide accordingly. If we are to support those with whom we work effectively then we must have the humility to accept what we do not know and to listen, hear and heed the voices of those who do.

PART ONE

The People and Their Needs

Introduction

The shuffling, drooling, long-stay psychiatric patient with regulation half-mast trousers; the 'mad axe murderer'; lazy; dangerous; stupid; romantic ideas of the mad artistic genius ... Many media portrayals of people who have serious mental health problems are as inaccurate as they are insulting. In our society those who experience such problems are often feared or looked down upon as a breed apart, not quite human.

In reality, the range of abilities present in people with mental health problems is no different from that of the population as a whole: mental illness does not respect intelligence or education. Those with serious mental health problems may have difficulties in the process of thinking or in using their abilities, but as the early Victorians recognized, thinking and intellect are not the same thing and mental health problems do not imply loss of intellect.

In the same way as a person in a wheelchair is not a child because they are unable to walk as adults are expected to do, someone with ongoing mental health problems is not a child because they have difficulty in concentrating on things or performing unaided all the basics of daily life. Neither are people with serious mental health problems lazy. The battle to balance the demands and expectations of an inner world, that no one else knows or understands, with those of the outside world, requires enormous determination (Hatfield, 1989). And this battle can be a very lonely affair, partly from an absence of friends and allies and partly from a lack of understanding on the part of others.

It is often very difficult for a person with serious mental health problems to explain their experiences to others, and for others to understand what they are saying. The words typically used to describe the experience of mental health problems – words like delusion, hallucination, flattening of affect, ideas of reference – were invented by people who had not themselves experienced the phenomena they were describing. They were invented by mental health professionals to describe what they saw in other people, and they are frequently arid descriptors of the phenomena they purport to describe. When someone's notes say that they have delusional beliefs this gives us very little information about that person's reality. Indeed, people with such difficulties are trying to describe things that are shared by no one else. Very few of us have experienced knowing that our nose controls the weather, or that all the food we eat is poisoned, or that the newscaster is controlling our thoughts. When people describe such experiences we typically adopt a kind of 'symptomatic reductionism' and declare the person to have a delusion or an idea of reference. By definition, this implies that what they are saying is 'not real' or 'not true' and needs no further exploration. It is all too frighteningly real and true for the person concerned.

The way in which we think about people who have serious ongoing mental health problems and their experiences is critical in determining our attitudes and behaviour towards them. If we think of someone as having a delusion we dismiss their experiences as unreal. If we consider them to be infantile we treat them like a child and do things for them, make decisions for them. If we construe someone as bad then we reprimand and admonish them. If we believe them to be lazy we chastise them and exhort them to make greater efforts. Most of all, if we believe the person to be mad then we disbelieve what they say. Can any of us say that we have never checked out what a client has told us with other staff? If someone says that they have been to Occupational Therapy, don't we frequently check it out with the Occupational Therapy department? Yet we almost never check out what a new member of staff tells us. What must it feel like when those who are helping us disbelieve us without corroborating evidence? If you are never believed then it is easy to cease to believe in yourself. As one young man said 'No one ever listens to what I say because I'm mad, empty, vague' (Perkins and Dilks, 1992, p. 5).

In Chapter 1 we explore the experience of serious mental health problems from the perspective of individuals with such difficulties and go on to look at ways in which the population as a whole might be defined. Chapter 2 identifies the underlying approaches most commonly used in relation to this client group. The problems and strengths of these models are discussed within the overall aim of promoting choice and autonomy for service users. In Chapter 3 we use the analogy of physical disability to argue that people who experience the cognitive and emotional problems characteristic of serious mental health difficulties might best be considered to be socially disabled. Someone with physical limitations is physically disabled because they are unable to negotiate the able-bodied physical world without help, support and adaptation of that world. Someone with cognitive and emotional problems is socially disabled because they are unable to negotiate the able-minded social world without help, support and adaptation of that world (Perkins and Dilks, 1992; Kitzinger and Perkins, 1993).

Ensuring access focuses not only, or even primarily, on changing the individual, but on changing the environment in which they function. It is within this context that the varying needs of people who are socially disabled might best be understood.

Understanding the people and their experiences | 1

Myriad diagnostic labels have been used to describe the difficulties of people with serious mental health problems. The most common diagnosis is that of schizophrenia, yet any population of seriously disabled service users typically includes some people with diagnoses of depression and manic-depressive illness, others with diagnoses of personality disorder, a few with anxiety-based problems, and some with organic problems such as Huntington's chorea and dementia. Unfortunately, these diagnoses tell us little about the individual or their personal reality: each is an umbrella term that includes many disparate experiences, needs and disabilities.

Many emotional and cognitive difficulties are not immediately obvious. Whereas it is usually evident that a person is blind or unable to walk, we cannot see that a person's thoughts are confused. We think that we know what it is like to be blind by closing our eyes, but we have great difficulty in even imagining what it is like not to be able to think properly, or to know that we are being poisoned when no one else believes us. However, we are able to gain some understanding of these experiences by listening to and reading people's own descriptions (for example, Hatfield, 1989; Perkins and Dilks, 1992; Deegan, 1993). Excerpts from these accounts are given here to offer a glimpse, a brief insight into the types of experiences with which such people live, but since everyone's experience is different, there is no substitute for talking to each person and exploring their individual world.

Some people find that they cannot think properly: their thoughts become confused and muddled:

> My thoughts get all jumbled up. I start thinking or talking about something and I never get there. Instead I wander off in the wrong direction and get caught up with all sorts of different things.

Torrey, 1983

Not being able to organize one's thoughts can be as frightening as it is disabling, as can problems of attention and concentration:

> If I am reading I may suddenly get bogged down at a word. It may be any word, even a simple word I know well. When this happens I can't get past it. It's as if I am seeing the word for the first time and in a much different way from anyone else. It's not so much that I am absorbed in it, it's more like it is absorbing me.

> *McGhie and Chapman, 1961*

Sometimes people experience altered sensations and perceptions – things look strange, different and very scary:

> Colours appear brighter, alluring almost, and my attention is drawn into the shadows, the lights, the intricate patterns of textures, the bold objects around me.

> *McGrath, 1984*

Or as one woman told us:

> Rachel, they're back, the air bubbles. At first I always believed they were part of every day, then you didn't know what I meant. I realised I was the only one who had them – bubbles hitting me all the time ... hitting me from every side, and my head is empty, empty as a shell, all of my thoughts drained out of me while I was asleep. All mixed up, day, night, whispers all around my head, lots of water, shoes don't seem to fit, colours, its all going on at once – it's killing me.

> Cited in *Kitzinger and Perkins, 1993*

Another experience is that of impaired identity – some people are unable to grasp quite who they are. As one extremely eloquent writer describes:

> Glassy shadows, polished pastels, a jigsaw puzzle of my body, face and clothes with pieces disappearing whenever I move. And if I want to reach out to touch me, I feel nothing but slippery coldness ... I know I am a 37-year-old woman, a sculptor, a writer, a worker, I live alone. I know all of this, but, like the reflection in the glass my existence seems undefined – more a mirage that I keep reaching for but never can touch.

> *McGrath, 1984*

Some people believe that strange things are happening: things different from what others believe, these are typically called 'delusions' or 'ideas of reference'. We have worked with someone who believed that she was about to be arrested and hanged for tax evasion. Another who believed she was receiving special messages making her do things from a particular newscaster on the television. Another who believed that he was responsible for the Vietnam war. It is easy to dismiss such implausible beliefs or regard them as totally ludicrous, yet they are a frightening reality for the person concerned. Their dilemma is often exacerbated by the fact that no one believes them. As one woman said to us:

> Not believing that I really feel, see or hear the things that trouble me – that's what makes me really lonely. People say things like 'don't worry', 'it's in your imagination', 'of course no-one is talking inside your head and at your ears', 'it's just not happening'. Well all I can say to that is 'Yes, it is happening, more's the pity', and 'yes it is difficult' – but they don't understand.

Many people's experiences of serious mental health problems are very frightening, quite unlike some more romantic accounts. However, it is important to remember that some people experience very profound and positive things. For example, one young man said to us:

> It was that day when I could see the whole of the universe spread out before me. I just stood there in the ward and I could feel it all. It was the most wonderful day of my life.

Or as another young woman said of her 'voices':

> Sometimes they're nasty about me – I don't like them then. But most of the time they're nice, they're funny, they keep me company – I'm not alone.

Whether a person's experiences are positive or negative, serious mental health problems often mean that the person has to balance their own, often scary internal world with that which others know. As one person said to us:

> My world is like having two or more different levels of what is right and what is wrong. Should I be pulling myself out to face the everyday motions of life there in your world? Having to keep it up is very difficult. I want to say slow down, have a rest, yet reality goes on and I feel as if I'm being smothered by life itself. My world hurts. It's never ending and painful. When I'm in my world I know I'm going far away, and although I know this, I can't prevent it. To me it's all so real, and I honestly believe it to be true and genuine when I'm there.

Cited in *Kitzinger and Perkins, 1993*

Another young man, who believed that people were trying to kill him, tried to explain to us the difficulty he experienced in refraining from attacking those whom he believed to have murderous intent:

> It's like when the telephone rings: you can ignore it for so long but eventually you just have to pick it up.

This analogy gives a vivid picture of his attempts not to act on his belief that people were going to attack him: of his efforts to hold on to others' reality and eventually succumbing to his own. How many times have we tried not to answer the telephone, but thought about how it could be something serious and eventually picked it up?

Frequently, serious mental health problems fluctuate leaving the person relatively well able to cope at some times and extremely distressed and disabled at others, seemingly unreliable and unpredictable to those around them, and frustrating to those who are trying to help them. Inevitably, these fluctuations pose difficulties for the person concerned:

> I can be fine for weeks, months sometimes, but I always have to live one day at a time. I plan things for next week, but I never believe that I will do them until the time arrives. I never know when they're going to come back – the voices, the ideas. That's the worst part. Knowing that they will come back but never knowing when.

These people who have written or spoken about their experience of serious mental health problems have told us a little of what their experiences might be like. Within this context we will now move on to look at some of the ways in which the population of people with serious ongoing mental health problems has been delineated by mental health professionals.

DEFINING THE POPULATION

People with serious ongoing mental health problems have been referred to by many names: 'chronically mentally ill', 'psychiatrically disabled' and 'long term mentally ill' to name but a few. There is controversy about the use of all of these terms. Not only does each refer to a diverse group of people with disparate strengths and problems, but the phrases themselves carry implicit value judgements that may be stigmatizing and self-fulfilling. In this book we have thus far used variants of the expression 'people with serious ongoing mental health problems' to describe those of us whose social functioning and ability to cope with the demands of day to day living is severely compromised as a consequence of cognitive and emotional problems.

As government policy in the UK and elsewhere demands that priority be accorded to those people with serious mental health problems (DOH, 1989a, 1990a, 1993a, 1994a), the issue of defining who this means becomes important. There is no consensus concerning such definitions (DOH, 1994b), but unless we can define who we are talking about further analyses of what we can do, and how to do it, are impossible.

Bachrach (1988) described three dimensions used to distinguish people with serious mental health problems: diagnosis, duration and disability. At the outset it is important to stress that these dimensions interrelate and that:

all three factors combine in defining enduring mental health problems so that no single factor is adequate. However taken separately they provide a useful framework for describing the population. (Bachrach, 1988, p. 384.)

We will begin, therefore, by critically examining each of these dimensions.

Diagnosis

Schizophrenia is the most common diagnosis in all groups of people with enduring mental health problems and several studies have shown that in excess of 50% of long term clients have such a diagnosis (Mann and Cree, 1976; Christie-Brown *et al.*, 1977; Ford *et al.*, 1995). Whether in hospital or the community, the effectiveness of care systems is therefore often judged in terms of their effectiveness for people with a diagnosis of schizophrenia. Indeed, Shepherd (1988) has gone so far as to suggest that if community services do not contain a majority of people with schizophrenia, then they are not providing for those who are most seriously disabled.

The preponderance of a diagnosis of schizophrenia amongst those with ongoing mental health problems has meant that most research attention has focused on this group. It has often been assumed that the services for those with a diagnosis of schizophrenia provide a model for all people with long term mental health problems. This is a mistake. There are many who are disabled by long term mental health problems who have different diagnoses. Numerous long term service users have affective disorders (depression or manic-depressive disorders). So called 'neurotic' problems can be at least as disabling as schizophrenia when, for example, a woman has been unable to leave her home unescorted for many years because of her agoraphobia, or must spend hours and hours engaged in the checking or cleaning rituals associated with obsessive/compulsive problems. Populations of long term service users also include people with organic problems, such as early dementias and Huntington's chorea.

In addition, many people who manifest an inability to cope with day to day life unaided have been diagnosed as suffering from 'borderline' or 'inadequate personality disorder': a sort of 'non-specific acopia', or inability to manage day to day life, in the absence of specific psychiatric symptomatology. These people are frequently rejected by the services they need because they are deemed not to have a mental illness (see Showalter, 1987; Wintersteen and Rapp, 1986). There is an interesting set of double standards in relation to 'personality disorder'. Whilst the Mental Health Act covers personality disorders (as well as mental illness and learning disabilities), it is not uncommon to find that community mental health services reject these people (Bachrach 1989; Hirsch *et al.*, 1992; Repper and Perkins, 1994). This issue is discussed further in the final section of this book.

Looking through the often extensive notes of people with ongoing mental health problems it is not uncommon to find that they have received numerous diagnoses over the years and have, in a manner of speaking, ended up with what appears to be a 'long-service' diagnosis of schizophrenia. The logic sometimes appears to be that if they have been in service care that long and are that disabled they must have schizophrenia. Further, many people with ongoing mental health problems have multiple diagnoses meaning that they cannot be placed neatly in any one diagnostic category. There has been increasing concern in the research and service literature about people with 'dual diagnosis', meaning those who have serious mental health problems and misuse drugs (Bachrach, 1988; Hirsch *et al.*, 1992).

Although diagnosis may be one way of describing people with long term mental health problems, it is not wholly satisfactory or sufficient. First, any one diagnosis encompasses a varied group of people. Second, no diagnosis predicts the exact course and outcome of the person's difficulties. For example, studies show that there are many people who have been diagnosed as having schizophrenia who do not experience ongoing disabilities. Birley (1991) in his review of long term outcome studies showed that only half of those with a diagnosis of schizophrenia had ongoing disability, and Summers and Hersch (1983) reported a similar level of disability in long term patients with a range of different diagnoses. Therefore, if a specific or circumscribed set of diagnoses is used to define a population in need of long term support two problems occur. On the one hand people may be included in services when they, in fact, do not need them. On the other hand they may be denied the services they need because they lack the requisite diagnosis. Diagnosis is not a good predictor of disability, support needs or as a condition of acceptance into a service.

In the light of these problems it is probably more useful to focus on the other dimensions outlined by Bachrach (1988): duration and disability.

Duration

Probably the most commonly used method of defining people with ongoing mental health problems is based on the duration of their contact with mental health services. People are deemed to have ongoing mental health problems because they either remain in hospital for long periods of time or have repeated readmissions to hospital.

With the development of community services many people with ongoing mental health problems can be supported in the community. As community services improve, so less use is made of hospital admission. If duration of hospitalization is used to define people with serious ongoing mental health problems, then it would spuriously appear that, with better community services, fewer people would have serious ongoing mental health problems. This would be a mistake and would detract attention from the intensive efforts of the better community services to maintain severely disabled people in their own communities. Therefore, in addition to length of hospitalization, considerations of duration now must include that group of people who have been in long term contact with community services.

The concepts of duration and type of contact have been used to describe three subgroups of the population with ongoing mental health problems: 'old long-stay', 'new long-stay' and 'new long term' clients (Wing and Morris, 1981). Although they are inevitably oversimplified, the distinction between these three groups can be useful in describing those people who have different histories and needs.

'Old long-stay' clients are those people who were admitted to hospital in the institutional era and who have lived there for many years, often most of their adult lives. The hospital has become their home, their entire world, and they have frequently grown old and frail there. For example, a study in the UK by Ford *et al.* (1987) found that 30% were aged over 75 years, 74% seldom left the hospital grounds and half of them rarely or never had visitors. Although the literature typically describes the old long-stay as a single group, there would seem to be grounds for differentiating subgroups within this population. Attempts to close hospitals have meant that an increasing number of old long-stay clients have been resettled, thus it appears useful to distinguish between resettled and hospitalized old long-stay groups.

The 'hospitalized old long-stay group' includes two broad subsets of people. First, there are those who, despite spending most of their lives in hospital, continue to manifest acute psychiatric symptomatology and behaviour problems that render them unacceptable in alternative facilities. On the other hand, there are those whose physical health problems (mobility, sight, hearing difficulties or dementia) mean that they require total nursing care. For example, one woman we know is 98 years old and has been in hospital for 70 years. She no longer manifests any psychiatric problems, but is blind and so frail that she cannot bear her own weight. She has to be fed, washed, dressed and is wheelchair bound. She appears to like being with familiar staff and does not respond to anyone she does not know, so she would be significantly disadvantaged if she were to be moved to a nursing home.

Those who have moved out of the hospital, the 'resettled old long-stay' group, typically require a high level of support and help in the community but frequently either no longer have acute symptomatology or their symptomatology does not interfere with their daily life. In short, their continuing needs are more similar to those of frail elderly people and they can often be accommodated in community facilities designed for this group.

'New long-stay' clients are those who, despite the development of community-based services, have not been able to remain in the community. They are that group of people who are currently being added to the old long-stay population. The experiences of this group are quite different from those of old long-stay clients. They began their psychiatric 'careers' in the post-institutional era and were often 'revolving door' clients – moving between hospital acute wards, home, and supported community accommodation before each of these finally rejected them and all that was left was a hospital long-stay facility. This group frequently manifest significant behaviour problems and continue to experience active symptomatology or a frequently fluctuating mental state. Unlike their old long-stay counterparts, they have often not been chronically 'institutionalized' and retain very normal ambitions. For example, despite being unacceptable even to general psychiatric hospital-based facilities because of their behaviour problems, all of the residents of a new long-stay facility where one of us works want a job, to get married and to have children. One young woman who has been hospitalized continuously for over a decade recently had a baby. The mean age of the residents of this unit is 32 years (all are under 34 years). On average they have been in contact with psychiatric services for 14.3 years and continuously hospitalized for 7.3 years (Perkins and Greville, 1993).

In a survey of 400 new long-stay patients in 15 hospitals, Mann and Cree (1976) found that 52% were female, most had a diagnosis of schizophrenia and some 16% had a severe physical disability. Although they constitute less than 7% of all hospital admissions, this group includes the most disabled individuals who currently present the greatest challenge to psychiatric services.

'New long term' clients differ from the previous two groups in that they do not stay in hospital for long periods of time, but they do make frequent use of a variety of services on a prolonged and repeated basis. The relative size of the new long term and new long-stay groups depends upon the extent and sophistication of community services. When better community services exist, the size of the long term group is increased. Where community services are relatively scarce, or rudimentary, fewer people with ongoing mental health problems can be supported in a community setting and the new long-stay population increases in size.

Although duration must, by definition, be a defining characteristic of that group of people with ongoing mental health problems, it is not without its difficulties. The criteria generally used to determine duration is length of contact with psychiatric services. This is problematic as it excludes two important groups of people. First, it excludes those who have ongoing mental health problems but never come into contact with psychiatric services, especially those who are homeless. Studies have shown that between 20 and 50% of homeless people have serious mental health problems (Gelberg and Linn, 1988; Timms and Fry, 1989; Weller, 1989) and contrary to popular belief these are not long-stay patients who have been discharged from mental hospitals after many years (Timms and Fry, 1989; Hirsch et al., 1992).

Second, it excludes that group of people who are never continuously in contact with services for long enough to be described as 'long term', although their problems and disabilities may well be enduring. Such people would benefit from support, but the fact that mental health services have frequently failed to form effective relationships with them, and the often compulsory nature of their contact with services, mean that they are often unwilling to avail themselves of this support: the services offered are unacceptable to them.

It is probably the case that duration of problems, rather than duration of contact with services, is the more important dimension to consider.

Disability

A disabilities approach was pioneered by Wing (1962), Wing and Brown (1970) and Wing and Morris (1981). This approach focuses on the concept of social disablement – a situation in which a person is unable to perform socially to the standards they expect of themselves, those expected by people important to them or by society in general. A person who is unable to perform socially to the standards they expect of themselves often experiences an acute sense of failure. In effect they have experienced a bereavement: a loss of the person they expected to be. It is a hard transition for anyone to move from undergraduate, or worker, to unemployed psychiatric patient. This sense of personal failure is compounded by the view of those important to the person: their opinion that the person has failed to live up to their expectations. It is difficult for parents, other relatives, friends and/or spouses, to come to terms with the person's disability and to accept, and more importantly to value, the person for what they are and not what they expected them to be. The situation is exacerbated by the popular images of madness portrayed in the media.

As Wing and Morris (1981) describe, this social disablement is a function not only of the symptoms of the person's mental health problems, but also of the ways in which they respond to these and of the social disadvantages that accrue. The potentially disabling symptoms associated with mental health problems include both what have been described as florid symptoms (delusion, hallucinations, ideas of reference) and negative symptoms (disturbances in thinking, concentration or emotional response, lethargy, lack of initiative). While these can be problematic, in and of themselves, they are not always disabling. For example, we know of one woman who talked almost continually to her 'voices' but was able to work as an audio typist for years: her work skills were not affected by her auditory hallucinations. Similarly, we know of a social worker who has 'a voice' and there are numerous people [including some of our colleagues and one of the present authors (REP)] who have periods when they are unable to work because of mental health problems, but after a period of sick leave are able to resume their former duties with no lasting problems.

These cognitive and emotional problems can lead to a person being particularly vulnerable to life events (see Falloon and Faddon, 1993) which others can take in their stride. For example, we knew one woman who lived in her own flat, receiving outreach support from psychiatric services: every time an electric bill arrived she became extremely distressed and disturbed (not infrequently requiring a brief hospital admission) even though she had the money to pay it.

One of the problems that often arises is that people with ongoing mental health problems, particularly those who are hospitalized, gradually do less and less. They cease to shop and cook for themselves, cease to go out, to work, to socialize and so forth. Such a gradual diminution of activity means that even appare: .y small tasks like going out to the pub or the shops become major undertakings – significant life events that can precipitate distress for someone who is particularly vulnerable. This can lead to a kind of vicious circle: if a person's symptoms worsen when they try what for them are new things (like going shopping) then there is a tendency to declare them unable to manage such activities, when with further experience the activity would become familiar and no longer distressing or disturbing.

It is these primary impairments that usually lead to diagnosis and treatment, but they are often not the reason for a person remaining in hospital or requiring support: the way in which the person responds to their experience of mental health problems and copes with their social disadvantages are frequently more important in this regard. Wing and Morris (1981) and Shepherd (1984) describe how dysfunctional responses to the experience of mental health problems typically take two forms.

Given prevailing societal views it is not surprising that many people find the idea of having mental health problems extremely frightening. It is tempting to cope with its occurrence by denying any problems at all. Such a reaction can be problematic: if the person considers that they have no problems then they may accept no help and therefore fail to make best use of their remaining abilities. In a recent study of referrals to the service in which one of us worked, one third of those people refusing to accept the service also considered that they had no mental health problems (Repper and Perkins, 1994).

At the other end of the spectrum, a person may be so frightened of exacerbating their problems and precipitating further relapse that they lose confidence entirely and avoid any stress or challenge. As this avoidance continues the person may become unwilling to do almost anything. Even the smallest everyday activities become a major challenge and withdrawal and apathy can result. Clearly, in such a situation the person may fail to make use of their remaining skills, abilities and interests.

Although these two types of reaction can be quite distinct, our experience suggests that it is not uncommon for any person to hold both perspectives simultaneously. In the hospital where one of us works, research has shown that some 50% of long-stay patients believe that they have not got, and never had, mental health problems (Taylor and Perkins, 1991), but at the same time, a substantial number believe themselves unable to do many things. In a recent conversation with one such client (who was at the time being closely observed) he said that there was nothing wrong with him and that he was going out to buy a car and visit his estranged wife with a view to their reconciliation. Later in the same conversation he talked about how much he needed the help of the staff because he couldn't do anything for himself any more and subsequently refused to go out to the shop saying that he was not up to it. Many people without mental health problems hold contradictory views simultaneously. How many people maintain that they cannot possibly sit another exam in their lives whilst planning their next course of study?

The ways in which a person copes with their mental health problems are not an intrinsic part of those difficulties, they are ordinary human responses to devastating life events. For example, many people told of their diagnosis of cancer refuse to believe it; Terry Waite (1993) writes of his endeavours to forget his captivity by going back to his past, only allowing himself to consider the implications of being held prisoner for short periods of time. Similarly, when someone we love dies, or we fail to get a job we want or we don't get the promotion we expected, it is not unusual to feel useless and hopeless. Denial and hopelessness are common reactions to unpleasant life events – and the experience of serious mental health problems can be a devastating life event.

The social disadvantages experienced by a person with ongoing mental health problems may predate these difficulties or result from them: they may have experienced a very poor and disrupted childhood. One woman we know had a mother who was an alcoholic and was continually being moved from her mother's home (where there were numerous 'uncles'), to foster homes and children's homes. By the age of 16, when her mother died, she had lived in 15 different places and each move had necessitated a change of school. Social disadvantages such as these, disrupted family relationships, poverty, poor education, even if not directly causal of mental health problems, leave a person with fewer personal and material resources with which to deal with the experience of mental health problems.

As well as pre-existing disadvantages that may handicap a person, numerous social disadvantages are meted out on those who experience serious mental health problems. Poverty is an important factor: those who are least able to cope with day to day life are expected to do so on the paltry income derived from state benefits on which most of us would fail to cope. In addition, there are many bars to activities and employment (in the services in which we work between 90 and 99% of long term service users are unemployed: Perkins and Greville, 1993; Repper and Perkins, 1995). Most importantly, the stigma associated with serious mental health problems is profoundly handicapping.

Studies of stigma show that it is highly related to continuing disability and accompanying demoralization (Gove, 1975). If you look odd, people avoid you in the street, will not sit next to you in the bus and disbelieve what you say. Not only is this demeaning, it can have other extremely deleterious consequences. For example, clinical experience suggests that, despite some excellent exceptions, complaints about physical ill health are not infrequently disbelieved by general hospital and general practice staff, meaning that the person does not get the physical health care they need.

Another problem experienced by those with serious ongoing problems is the contrast between their own situation and that of the staff who help them. As nurses and direct care staff are often the most accessible to the client, it is they who most frequently experience the anger that this contrast predictably engenders. The social isolation of many people with ongoing mental health problems means that sometimes nurses and direct-care staff are the only people with whom they have an ongoing relationship, and these staff have everything their clients want: a job, status, money, a home, a car, relationship, families, friends ... This situation was graphically illustrated by one young man who, very angry, burst into a staff meeting and said 'You're all fucking paradise people!' In response to such anger it is often tempting to respond by outlining how poor we are, but this is a mistake. It is far more appropriate to express a sympathy for the person's appropriate anger at the poverty that accompanies mental health problems and help them to direct it in a more appropriate direction. For example, a group of clients with whom one of us works are in regular correspondence with their MP and the staff who work with them often lend their support by signing the letters as well.

Aims of interventions and approaches to care

2

Before we can help anyone in any situation it is necessary to decide what that help is designed to achieve. As with any journey, we cannot decide on the best route or mode of transport until we have talked at length with the person we are going with and have agreed some destination. With help, people with serious disabilities are usually able to identify many goals. They might want to get out of hospital, be more independent, get rid of their symptoms, have a girl/boyfriend, get a job or make more friends, have a baby or feel less isolated. Although these may all be laudable aspirations, sometimes it may not be possible to address everything a person wants to do at once. We may therefore have to help people choose what is most important for them.

For example, a 38 year old woman with whom we work lives in a staffed house in the community, values her work in open employment and regularly visits the local bingo hall and friends in the area. However, she does little in the way of housework, laundry, shopping or cooking. Considerable efforts to increase her skills in these areas have enabled her to perform these activities independently, but they are time consuming. This leaves her no time to pursue her evening leisure activities and makes her late for work in the morning, thus jeopardizing her employment. If her aim were to become more independent and live in a more normal setting then we might resettle her in a flat of her own, but this would jeopardize the work and leisure roles that are important to her. If her main interests are her work and leisure activities then she may have to remain in some form of sheltered living situation where she can be relieved of domestic chores. In short, she may have to choose between having her own home and maintaining her work and leisure activities.

Often different professionals in the same team will hold differing opinions about the decisions that should be made in such situations, and of course there are no right answers. Increasing independence, for example, is not in any absolute terms 'better' than increasing access to normal social roles and activities.

We firmly believe that the best way of proceeding is to let the individual concerned be the judge of what is most important for him/her.

Decisions about the aims of support are important but we also need a model to guide us. The models we use determine our understanding of the person's problems and leads us to different priorities and interventions. For example, if we adopt a wholly medical model then we will only assess symptoms; if we adopt a skills-based model we will assess a person's competencies and train them. The model we use also determines the type of interventions we adopt, the ways in which we judge success and ultimately the morale of both staff and clients.

CURE-BASED APPROACHES

Notions about cure pervade most health care, including mental health services. Cure-based models are not limited to the 'medical model': they permeate most of our professional training. Most professionals learned how to identify a person's 'symptoms', whether these are seen in terms of neurochemical imbalances, faulty cognitions, disturbed intra-psychic processes or dysfunctional family relationships. Training then focuses on a plethora of interventions aimed to put things right – medication, psychotherapy, family therapy, cognitive therapy, counselling, advice ... – the list of different types of interventions in both mainstream and complementary areas is almost endless. All of these cure-based approaches focus upon identification of underlying problems and interventions to remove them.

Such 'cure' models are of limited utility in work with people who have ongoing disabilities. First, people whose problems are ongoing have usually experienced numerous cure-based interventions and their difficulties remain. Continuing to adopt cure-based approaches can be positively damaging to both clients and staff because of the demoralization and hopelessness that results when a 'cure' cannot be effected. If we expect to eliminate someone's symptoms and we cannot then we feel like failures, and we may become demoralized or find ourselves blaming our failures on the shortcomings of the people we work with. But more importantly, if we raise our clients' expectations of cure, then they will feel hopeless and useless when they experience yet another relapse: it is not uncommon for people to feel guilty and blame themselves when treatment does not work.

It is never easy to accept disability whether it be physical or social, many people spend large amounts of time and money seeking cures for both physical and social disabilities. A focus of cure as the only solution and the only way that a person can have a meaningful and happy life has the negative effect of implying that life with disability is not worth living. Thus, someone who has lost the use of their legs, is unable to hear or see, or has thinking or concentration difficulties is somehow a lesser being and their life cannot be satisfying and worth while. Our desire to believe that all problems can be put right is oppressive of those who are disabled.

Cure-based models have also led to a prioritization of treatment and a devaluing of support and care. Treatment or specific therapy of some kind has a higher status within most of our services than does helping someone with day to day tasks like bathing and cleaning, or supporting someone in doing the things they want to do. It seems that the status accorded to treatment has led to many ordinary activities receiving 'treatment' labels. We no longer talk to someone, we do 'counselling', activities such as doing the gardening become occupational therapy, gardening therapy, work therapy. Other activities are described in spuriously technical terms not in common usage: bathing becomes 'self-care' and cleaning one's room becomes 'home management'.

Support is important in its own right and it is not helpful to label every activity of life a therapy, because once it becomes a therapy it is rendered abnormal, removed from everyday life and experience. If the aim of our interventions is to help people with disabilities to have access to normal activities and roles, then calling this support and help 'therapy' – which is typically a time-limited affair – is not useful. Often we declare an intervention not to have 'worked' if, when the support stops, the problems have not gone away or they recur. If a person's problems are ongoing then support will often need to be ongoing as well, and the fact that it is ongoing is not a failure.

SKILLS-BASED APPROACHES

Ideas about developing skills and skills training are very popular in many services for people with serious ongoing mental health problems. This type of approach (see Anthony and Margules, 1974; Anthony, 1977, 1979) starts by identifying a person's skills and skills deficits. The things that it is necessary for a person to learn are then broken down into their component parts and intervention takes the form of building-up competency largely within a behavioural framework.

This type of approach helps interventions to be systematic and organized. It also offers a clear direction for work: once a skills deficit has been identified skills training is employed to develop that area of functioning. Rehabilitation is often seen as synonymous with skills training and development, usually with a view to resettlement and discharge once a sufficient repertoire of skills have been developed. But this perspective is fraught with problems.

If acquiring the ability to independently perform a satisfactory repertoire of skills is seen as a condition for 'discharge into the community' then many people will remain in institutions. Ongoing disability often means that continuing support, rather than time-limited training, is necessary to maintain skilled performance. A focus on training actively mitigates against ensuring access to communities – this requires the provision of support and environmental adaptations.

If a certain skills repertoire is necessary for community living then this implies that the disabled individual has to be rendered suitable for the community, rather than that community rendered suitable for them. The concept of 'access' as it applies to physically disabled individuals involves changing the community at least as much as changing the individual. A person without legs may be taught how to use a wheelchair, but thereafter all adaptations are down to the community, e.g. ramps, lifts, wide doors, sloped curbstones for crossing roads, lowered work surfaces, etc. If people who are socially disabled by ongoing thinking and feeling problems are to have similar rights of access then the focus must be on supports and adaptations of the environment as well as upon changing the individual.

A skills-based approach can only be used when there is an identifiable skill that can be taught. This may be reasonable in relation to basic mechanical skills, like cleaning one's teeth or using public transport, but it becomes less so when one moves on to social and emotional areas. Although many people with ongoing mental health problems have social difficulties, social skills training, despite its popularity, has shortcomings (Shepherd, 1977, 1978). There is a widely recognized 'generalization problem' in social skills training: something learned in one setting often does not change behaviour in other settings. Social competence, for example, requires far more than the acquisition of simple behavioural tasks: it is necessary to judge what behaviour is required in any situation and then continually change behaviour on the basis of the feedback we get from others.

Skills training approaches typically ignore the cognitive components of skilled performance. These components are obvious in social areas but are also central in many apparently mechanical tasks. Even in the area of cooking or bathing the goal is rarely to enable to person to cook a meal or have a bath: more commonly the aim is for the person to organize their nutritional requirements or keep themselves acceptably clean. These latter endeavours involve many cognitive judgemental and organizational skills. For example, planning what food to buy on the basis of what we have in our cupboards and who is coming to see us, deciding what we fancy eating, when to buy it and what to get if the things we want are not available, not to mention remembering that the shops might be closed on Sundays and Bank Holidays and adjusting our schedule. Most people, most of the time, are unaware of making these type of judgements – they become automatic, like driving a car. But most people who drive will also remember how impossible the task felt when they started: trying to steer, change gear, deciding where to go and avoiding other road users all at the same time! In this area a focus on skills training fails to acknowledge the nature of the difficulties experienced by people with ongoing mental health problems. Many experience specific thinking and concentration difficulties that make the cognitive demands of even basic tasks difficult.

Old long-stay hospital residents who have been institutionalized for many years may have been denied the opportunities of practising a great many skills (such as shopping, cooking, cleaning) and may require opportunities and help to do these things again. It is not uncommon for things to have changed since they were last outside hospital. Many residents will only know about buses that have conductors, or money that came in pounds, shillings and pence. However, for those who have not been institutionalized, it is rarely the mechanical skills with which they experience difficulties, but the cognitive components of skilled performance. In this context it is worth remembering that there are alternatives to doing it yourself in many areas. Take-aways, cafés and service washes at launderettes can all be handy, and having someone do your cleaning for you is not abnormal.

Skills training is of extremely limited utility in emotional and psychological areas. The way a person responds to and copes with the experience of ongoing mental health problems is very important (Wing and Morris, 1981; Shepherd, 1984; Taylor and Perkins, 1991; Perkins and Moodley, 1993a). Adapting to the experience of serious ongoing mental health problems is a bereavement process: lamenting the loss of a life that one had or expected to have and coping with the challenge of building life afresh in a society where one is stigmatized and often excluded. The way in which a person copes and adapts is of central importance in determining the extent to which they are able to use their abilities, but the skills approach can contribute little in this regard. The absence of skills must not be confused with the inability to use them, and the latter is far more common.

A skills approach can lead to the inappropriate prioritization of interventions: it tends to focus attention on those areas where there is an identifiable skill that can be learned. Not infrequently this leads to a mismatch between the things that the client and staff consider important. The client may want help to feel better, to get a new flat, to get more money; the staff, feeling unable to provide such things, try to turn the person's attention to their budgeting and self-care and attempt to distract them from that which is distressing them.

It is sometimes argued that skills training has the advantage of adopting an educational approach where the client takes on the valued role of student and the staff are the instructors and facilitators. Whilst the status of undergraduate, medical student or nursing student may be valued, the skills training that occurs within psychiatric services can hardly be seen as a parallel. When the skills being taught are ones that it is assumed that all adults have, it can be very demeaning and infantalizing for the person, a problem experienced in other areas, such as adult literacy. Imagine what it would feel like to you, an adult, to be taught to clean your teeth, or boil an egg ... as one client said to us 'I'm not going to that class again – they talk to me like I used to talk to my son when he was little. I'm not a kid, you know.'

The relative roles in a skills-training approach where the member of staff is the trainer and the client is the pupil, or trainee, automatically devalue the client as learner – the one without skills – and value the staff as teacher – the one with skills. If we are to value those whom we serve then this relationship must be

changed. Some people will need help with day to day activities, but how different the situation would be if we adopted the model that non-disabled people
have with their helpers. Many people get help and support from cleaners, cafés,
service washes, but, in every case, the person getting the help is in charge, says
how they want things done ... How different our services would look if this
principle were applied to the sorts of help given by staff to those disabled by
mental health problems. At the very least, being with and doing with should
take precedence over instructing and observing and are much more conducive to
the formation of good therapeutic relationships.

NEEDS APPROACHES

Probably the most popular idea in mental health services is that of needs:
frequently questions are asked about the nature and extent of service users'
needs and the degree to which services meet those needs. Throughout the literature on long term care, many writers have talked about needs (Wing and
Morris, 1981; Bennett, 1978, 1980; Shepherd, 1984) and have developed ways
of assessing needs (for example, Brewin *et al.*, 1987, 1988). These models
essentially move away from symptoms and skills deficits to a consideration of
the complex requirements of each individual. Such approaches also allow
consideration of a range of ways in which an individual's needs can be met.
Instead of restricting the focus to symptom removal or skills training, once a
person's needs have been identified a variety of ways to meet them can be
tailored to the individual's needs. The destructive failure inherent in cure and
skills perspectives can be avoided. For example, if a person is unable to manage
domestic chores there are numerous ways in which their domestic needs can be
met including home helps and cleaners.

Despite the prevalence and popularity of a needs-based approach, there are
enormous problems with it, most of which centre around the question 'What is
a need?' On the one hand, the term 'need' has been used to refer to everything
from basic physiological necessities (food and warmth) to complex psychological needs such as esteem and belonging. On the other hand, mental health
services often think about needs in terms of service inputs: need for a day
centre, need for hospitalization or need for medication (for example, Brewin *et
al.*, 1987, 1988). These two uses have become confused so that the need for
nutrition is considered in the same manner as the need for a group home, when
the two are self-evidently quite different. Nutrition is basic to human life, a
group home is simply one way of organizing services to ensure that those needs
basic to human life are met.

There is very little clarity about what constitutes a 'need' in the field of
mental health and many of the confusions revolve around the question of who
decides what a person's needs are. Numerous day to day examples of this exist
within our services. For example, a client may define themselves as needing to

be allowed to lie in bed late in the morning because they feel tired. Staff, aware of some of the detrimental effects of doing nothing (Wing and Brown, 1970), say that the person needs to get up. Whose opinion should take precedence?

There are many 'interested parties' who define the needs of individuals: mental health professionals, other carers, friends, family, general practitioners, courts, police, other people who use mental health services, society at large, mental health pressure groups, service-user organizations, as well as the individual whose needs are being defined. Too often it is assumed that there can be some consensus reached between all of these groups and individuals when the reality is that their agendas and interests are often at odds with each other.

Any definition of 'need' inevitably involves political and ethical judgements: whereas a civil rights position might claim that people with ongoing mental health problems have a right to be part of communities, a paternalistic perspective might argue that there is a duty to protect those who are vulnerable from themselves and from potentially harmful situations. In extreme cases, the law and Mental Health Act specify certain boundaries, but these are of little help in most instances where decisions have to be made between a duty of care, the individual's freedom and liberty, the wishes of relatives and the protestations of neighbours.

We have already argued that, wherever possible, the individual's wishes should be paramount, and we would maintain this position here. At the bottom line, where differences of opinion exist our primary task is to enable the disabled person to achieve what they want to achieve. This does not mean we ride roughshod over the views and concerns of relatives, neighbours and others, rather that we work with them, and support them, in enabling the disabled person to achieve his/her ambitions.

Unfortunately, much needs assessment in mental health services is still designed to evaluate needs for specific supported accommodation, work, day activity and treatment. When we look at the 'needs' of long-stay hospital residents we are generally looking at whether they need high-staffed accommodation or low-staffed accommodation, or nursing homes (Brewin et al., 1987, 1988; Clifford, 1989). Whilst such assessments may be useful in an attempt to close hospitals they are dangerous for two reasons.

First, they tend to create this special breed of human being – the mental patient – who has needs that are quite different from those of the rest of the population. Nobody actually needs a day centre or a hostel or a hospital, these are simply ways that have been developed to ensure that ordinary human needs for shelter, occupation or safety are met. People with serious ongoing mental health problems have exactly the same needs as everyone else. The difference lies in the resources and abilities that they have to meet these needs. As we have already seen, those who experience serious ongoing mental health problems are not only disabled by the cognitive and emotional difficulties that these bring, but also by social disadvantages: lack of material and social resources on which most people rely so heavily, and the stigma and exclusion that being a 'mental patient' so often brings. These factors all conspire to ensure that a person's needs are not met. This does not mean that the individual is in some way stupid or incompetent, merely that they are often deprived of those things necessary to ensure that their needs are met: colleagues, friends, work, home, family, financial, personal and material resources. Hospitals, hostels, day centres and the like, are a substitute – often a poor one – for the absence of these other supports.

The second problem is that defining needs in relation to facilities and services available mitigates against new and innovative means by which a person can be helped. For example, if someone is unable to meet their nutritional requirements unaided then it is often assumed that they need to live in a special sheltered setting where meals are provided: a hostel or staffed house, or sometimes even a hospital. This has the side effects of ghettoization and depriving the person of a home of their own. There are many other ways in which nutritional requirements can be met but sometimes these have to be creatively tailored to the individual's requirements. We know of one man who had his 'meals on wheels' delivered to the pub where he spent his lunch times, this being the only way to ensure that he got them. Despite a desire to develop a needs-led service, if needs are defined in terms of specific facilities then what results is that very resource-led service, from which we are trying to depart: a person's needs being defined in terms of the resources that are available.

One way of thinking about needs that has proved useful in a mental health setting is that put forward by Maslow (1970). He argued that the human needs should be thought of as a hierarchy: that the satisfaction of those needs at the bottom of the hierarchy (basic physiological needs) is a prerequisite for satisfaction of those at higher levels. For example, if a person is starving or suffocating then needs for love, sex, status and even personal safety take second place to the acquisition of food or oxygen. The hierarchy he defined comprised of five levels:

- Physiological needs include the need for oxygen, food, water – all the things that are necessary for the normal homeostasis of the body.
- Needs for personal safety and a safe environment include physical and emotional security and the need for a safe place to live.
- Needs for love, affection and belonging include needs for warmth, interest and encouragement from others together with a sense of belonging.
- Needs for esteem include the need for respect, acknowledgement and recognition from others, self-respect, competence, confidence – the need for being valued and valuing oneself.
- Need for self-actualization refers to the acceptance of oneself and others for what we/they are.

Amongst people with serious ongoing mental health problems many of these needs are not met by the facilities and services offered. For example, it is commonly argued that hospitals offer a place of safety yet many people who have been admitted to hospital have been threatened, attacked and/or robbed whilst there, and sexual harassment and assault are all too common (see Gorman, 1992). Among the residents on units for those who have serious ongoing mental health problems where one of us works, some 80% reported having been physically assaulted within the last year (Perkins and Greville, 1993). Living in a sheltered community facility or attending a day centre may offer a sense of belonging but it probably does little to enhance a person's self-esteem or sense of self-worth. In a survey of the opinions of service users, Estroff (1993) found that many of their needs remained unmet and inadequately addressed by services. The most commonly occurring unmet needs identified by services users were for an adequate income, intimacy and privacy, a satisfying sexual life, meaningful work, a satisfying social life, happiness, adequate resources and warmth.

It is important to note that these are all ordinary, human needs, common to everyone. It may be difficult to define what a need is, but it remains the case that the needs of people with serious mental health problems are the same as those of everyone else. The difference is that clients' needs often remain unmet. At the level of both individual care planning and service development, our task is to ensure access to those relationships, facilities and activities that will enable a person to meet their needs. That is, providing the necessary support and shelter to enable these socially disabled individuals to have access to the ordinary social world and to become valued members of our societies.

There have been some famous people who have experienced serious mental health problems – artists, musicians, painters, etc. – and who have achieved a highly respected status in society (for example, John Ogden, Leonardo da Vinci). However, most of us, whether or not we have serious mental health problems, do not have outstanding talents. Access for those who are socially disabled by ongoing mental health problems cannot be contingent upon special gifts: it must be a right accorded to them as citizens. In the context of ensuring that an individual's needs are met, we will now explore further these ideas about social disability and access.

3

Social disability and access

Ideas about social disability in relation to serious ongoing mental health problems have been developed from the work of Wing and his colleagues (1962, 1970, 1981). They conceptualized social disablement as the situation in which a person is unable to perform socially to the standards they expect of themselves and that others expect of them. It is clear from Wing and Morris's (1981) discussion of those factors that contribute to 'social disablement' that disability results as much from the way in which society treats a person with serious mental health problems as from their emotional and cognitive problems. It is also clear that the extent to which a person is handicapped by their emotional or cognitive limitations is in large part determined by the social conditions and expectations that prevail.

This work takes a much broader view of the individual than the exclusively medical model: it moves away from a focus on diagnosis by including consideration of the social disadvantages which contributed to their handicap. At a descriptive level, this model is useful in encouraging a perspective that looks beyond psychiatric symptoms and takes account of the individual's responses and coping mechanisms as well as their social situation, and the way in which these interact. However, at an analytical level, it does not move beyond a description of disability. It tends to lead to defining a person as a long list of problems: an inaccurately negative and demoralizing view of the person concerned. It gives those trying to help no indication of where they should start or what they should do.

Many people with serious ongoing mental health problems have multiple disabilities, but they are not universally disabled. Everyone has some qualities and talents and these become central if we extend the model developed by Wing and Morris (1981) and think not about social disability alone, but also about access in a manner that parallels consideration of access for people who are physically disabled.

A person who experiences physical limitations is unable to negotiate the 'normal' (able-bodied) physical world without support, help and adaptation of that world. The handicap that someone with mobility problems experiences is far greater in the absence of such adaptations as ramps, mobility aids, wide doorways, transport and lifts which give them access to roles, activities and facilities within our communities. We have argued that people with the cognitive and emotional problems associated with serious ongoing mental health problems might best be considered to be socially disabled: unable to negotiate the 'normal' (able-minded) social world without help, support and adaptation of that world. Whilst that social world is beginning to consider issues of access for people with physical limitations there has been scant attention to what access might mean for those who are socially disabled by cognitive and emotional limitations. Whether a person is physically or socially disabled the purpose of supports and adaptations that ensure access is to enable them to use their skills and abilities and to live the life they want to lead.

Our basic premise is that work with people who experience serious ongoing mental health problems – socially disabled people – should be directed towards ensuring that they have access to the social world: access to ordinary social facilities, roles, relationships and activities. These are the roles and activities to which most people in our society have access and through which their needs, at all levels, are met. They are also the roles and activities from which socially disabled people are often excluded. It is only by ensuring such access that we can hope to ensure that they are able to meet their needs. It is not the role of staff to meet the needs of the clients but to ensure that clients have the opportunity to meet their own needs.

Within the field of physical disability, as well as in the mental health area, there have been numerous discussions about the term 'disability'. Some have argued that we should use terms with more positive connotations such as 'challenged' or 'differently able'. We believe that there are serious problems with using such alternatives. The term 'challenged' underplays the extent of people's difficulties by implying that they could be just like everybody else if they 'rose to the challenge'. Of course, the converse of this is that people who continue to have problems have simply not tried hard enough – they have failed to rise to the challenge. Ongoing mental health problems cause serious difficulties and the idea that they could rise to the challenge of 'normality' if they just tried hard enough is cruel and oppressive.

The term 'differently able' also minimizes the impact of problems. We are not arguing that people with serious ongoing mental health problems have no abilities. Far from it. Such people have the same range of abilities and skills as those who are not disabled. However, their ability to use these skills is impaired by their problems. Serious ongoing mental health problems often have a devastating effect on people's lives: a fact that is not recognized if we simply assume that they have different abilities. Our use of the idea of social disability is intended to highlight both the involuntary nature of the disability, and thus avoid oppressive victim blaming, and highlight the need for social changes within our communities to accommodate it (Kitzinger and Perkins, 1993). As we have seen, a great many of the problems experienced by those with serious mental health problems are a consequence of the way in which our society treats people with such difficulties. The model of social disability and access that we have outlined here has several important implications.

1. **The person is central: their interests and preferences as well as their social circumstances.** It is not possible to ensure access without determining access to what – and this will differ from individual to individual. For some access to a work role may be central. For others, access to domestic or family roles may be paramount. Often it is argued that people with serious ongoing mental health problems are unrealistic in wanting what most people in our society take for granted. To declare someone to be unrealistic is to allow us to ignore what they want. It is our contention that when a person is deemed unrealistic what we are really saying is that we lack the ingenuity or the resources to help them to achieve what they want. This change from defining the person as at fault (unrealistic) to defining us and our services as failing (lacking ingenuity and resources) is an important shift in focus. The responsibility lies with us: it may not be an individual failing on our part, but nevertheless we have failed those whom we serve. Even with inadequate resources there are ingenious ways in which someone can be helped to achieve what they want, or at least a close approximation to it. Examples from our own experience include: a woman who badly wanted a home of her own but found it difficult to organize her day to day life without someone around to help. She was provided with befrienders paid to live in her house and offer her the help she needed. A woman who wanted a job, but was extremely disruptive in a work setting, was helped to organize outwork knitting which she could do at home.

   If we are really unable to provide the person with the help necessary to achieve their ambitions, then we can tell them the realities of the situation: not that they are unrealistic, but that we have not got the resources.

2. **A range of different interventions, supports and strategies can be utilized.** A disabilities model does not require that we choose between a medical or psychological or social approach to help the person achieve access to those activities, relationships and facilities that they desire – any of these might be used. Some people may be helped by taking medication to reduce symptomatology that is impeding their progress. Others may be helped by acquiring particular skills. Yet others by having someone to talk to in a more informal manner about their hopes and fears, or someone to go and do things with them. Others might need practical help or someone to do some things for them so that their time and energies are released for activities that are more important to them. This kind of trade-off is not uncommon and one which many people make all the time. How many of us are relieved of cooking (by going out for a meal or getting a take-away) so that we have time to do something else that is important to us?

   There is often an unhelpful moralizing that pervades our work with people who experience serious mental health problems: basic activities of life take precedence over pleasure and leisure. Unless the person has cleaned, ironed and washed their socks they should not go to the pub. Indeed, in a recent talk one of us was asked by a service manager where rehabilitation stopped and pleasure started: health services in her view are not about giving people pleasure. A person who is socially disabled by definition has difficulty in performing things expected of them: this is why they need support. If we are really to help to enhance the individual's quality of life then this kind of moralizing is unhelpful. We may need to relieve a person of some tasks that have little meaning for them in order to help them to engage in those roles that really do enhance their self-worth and quality of life. Of course, individuals differ in this regard. Some people would rather be a home-maker than a worker, others derive their status, contacts and self-worth from their work. The question that each of us should ask ourselves is, if we were seriously disabled, which roles would we give up in order to least threaten our esteem, status and worth?

It is important to remember that it is not always staff who have the expertise necessary to help someone achieve those things that are important to them. Frequently, someone who has been in the situation and knows what it is like – someone with the expertise of experience – is a more useful ally and supporter. This premise is the one on which most self-help organizations are based: other service users have a wealth of expertise that can be useful to others in the same position.

3. **The focus shifts from changing the disabled individual to changing the society.** This involves providing prosthetic aids and support that parallel the wheelchair for someone with mobility problems or the signer for someone with hearing impairment. Clearly, a person may want to develop their skills but in many situations achieving access involves changing the expectations of the situation to accommodate them. None of us would want always to have to change to fit in: we want to be accepted as we are. Sometimes this can mean simple practical assistance like providing transport or someone to go with you to help you negotiate new situations. All of us know how difficult this can be. Even something as simple as a café presents problems: do we sit down and wait to be served or do we go to the counter and order? Do we wait at the counter for our food or sit at the table and it will be brought to us? Do we pay when we receive our food or when we have finished? Do we leave a tip or is it included? The situation is even more difficult if we are in a foreign country, but we must remember that for many people who are socially disabled, especially those who have lived in hospital or other sheltered settings for some time, the world that seems so ordinary to us resembles a foreign country. If the person experiences the cognitive and emotional problems associated with ongoing mental health problems then it can be doubly difficult without someone to help.

Whilst practical assistance and changes can be important, access to the social world essentially involves access to ordinary social roles (worker, friend, father, golfer). It is to our advantage that roles are not simply defined by sets of rules and expectations: roles are relational (Shepherd, 1984). They are negotiated between the people involved. There is no set of skills that defines a worker – the role of worker differs from job to job. Many families have different arrangements about the roles of the partners involved; different friendships operate in different ways; sexual relationships can be many and varied. As roles are negotiated between those involved they can be renegotiated and often some change in expectations can enable a socially disabled person to have access to roles that would otherwise be denied them. Much work with families, neighbours, friends, employers and others in the community can usefully be seen as the renegotiating of roles. In a work setting, for example, it may be possible to change the expectations upon a person in order to enable them to perform the job. For example, we have already mentioned a woman who worked as a typist despite hearing voices with which she conversed with most of the time. Whilst these voices did not affect her competency she did disturb the work of others where she worked. In negotiation with the employer she was moved to a small unused side office where she did not disturb people and she was able to continue in employment.

Often people with serious ongoing problems have existing social networks who want to offer support but find it difficult to cope with their friends' problems. Disabled people often describe their friends gradually drifting away because they did not understand and did not know what to do. This drift can be avoided if the person can be helped to maintain contact. One young gay man who we know had a quite extensive network of people who came to his flat and looked after him. This raised problems in two ways. The young man himself got fed up with someone being there all the time to look after him and this way of helping was extremely taxing on the time and resources of his friends. With the approval of the man himself, a meeting was held in which these problems were considered. The ensuing discussion resulted in a plan in which the social time that he spent with his friends increased and the amount of practical help decreased, some of this help being transferred to statutory services in order to preserve the friendship network.

Much family work (see Smith and Birchwood, 1990; Tarrier, 1992) can be seen as changing expectations within the family. This can involve helping them to understand the possibilities and problems of someone with social disabilities: what they find difficult and, equally importantly, the skills that they have, things that exacerbate their difficulties and ways in which the family can include them, and what ongoing support all involved will need. There is much consideration of 'the burden of care on the family' – an extremely devaluing way of describing a disabled individual and one which completely ignores the burden of the family on the disabled individual. Being cared for can be an enormous burden and it is usually easier to give help than receive it. Accepting help makes one feel incompetent, guilty, as well as imposing the burden of behaving in the way our carer wants and being suitably grateful even though we did not want to need the help in the first place.

Considering access for people who are socially disabled essentially means focusing on their strengths and interests. That is, enabling a person to make the best use of their strengths and pursue their interests by providing that support and help which is necessary to minimize the disruptive consequences of their problems. We cannot value a socially disabled person unless we are able to recognize their strengths, we cannot build a good working relationship with someone whom we see as having no assets, no value. We cannot facilitate their valuing of themselves without a recognition of their abilities and we cannot help them to meet their needs effectively unless we can identify the resources and talents that they have.

All too often the way in which we think and talk about socially disabled people revolves around their problems: their symptoms, behavioural disturbance and the things they cannot do. If the help we offer revolves primarily around problems then we get into a vicious cycle of hopelessness. Such hopelessness means that the person becomes increasingly discouraged and disinclined to persist with whatever they are doing. Everyone knows that when we are continually criticized about the things we are doing we tend to give up. On the other hand, if others focus on the things we are doing well, then we are inclined to persist and make greater efforts buoyed by the pleasure of success. Our clients are no different from ourselves. In considering access for socially disabled people we are not saying that a person's problems are completely unimportant rather that they take second place to their strengths, interests and assets.

TREATMENT, SUPPORT AND SHELTER

Within the social disability and access model that we have described, any treatment or intervention must be judged in terms of the extent to which it facilitates access to roles, relationships and activities that are valuable to the person concerned. In this context it is important to draw a distinction between treatment, support and shelter.

Treatment refers to those pharmacological and psychological interventions that are designed to decrease or remove a person's cognitive and emotional problems. It is undoubtedly the case that some of these can be helpful, but, as we have seen, they cannot form the sole basis of work with those who are socially disabled by ongoing cognitive and emotional problems. Indeed, Shepherd (1984) argued that treatment was essentially part of the assessment process, defining the limits of disability: see what problems you can't get rid of and work out ways of helping the disabled person live with those that are left. Support and shelter are important ways of minimizing the disruptive effects of problems that cannot be removed. In general, support in ordinary situations should take precedence over the provision of shelter, but sheltered environments still have a role to play in our services.

Support refers to any help that we give someone to enable them to engage in an activity or occupy a role. In relation to physical disability this may refer to the provision of mobility aids and adaptations of the able-bodied physical environment to facilitate access. In relation to social disability it refers to the provision of help and adaptations that render the able-minded social world accessible. We have discussed how this might include a variety of forms of help and renegotiation of roles and expectations of the 'ordinary' (able-minded) world.

Shelter, on the other hand, refers to the creation of special environments for the disabled person. In relation to both physical and social disability this might include a range of special supported living, work and leisure situations. Instead of offering support in an 'ordinary' setting, a separate facility is provided.

In general, the tendency has been to provide socially disabled people with shelter in the form of hostels, group homes, supported houses, sheltered workshops, leisure and social groups, day centres and clubs. Many of these have played an important role in decreasing reliance on that ultimate and total sheltered living situation, the psychiatric hospital. However, there is now a trend away from the provision of shelter towards giving people a higher level of support in ordinary settings through intensive outreach schemes. There are many advantages of providing support to ensure access to roles, relationships, activities and facilities that already exist within communities (Test and Stein, 1978; Hoult, 1986; Rapp and Wintersteen, 1989; Ford et al., 1995). First, these communities offer a wealth of opportunities – a range much greater than is possible in sheltered provision. Second, the use of ordinary community facilities helps to break down the divisions between those who have been defined 'mad' and those who have not. It is only by breaking down these barriers, and ensuring that people with social disabilities have the opportunity to engage in the full range of relationships and activities that our society affords, that we can truly say that socially disabled people have the rights of access that all citizens reasonably expect. Third, it is generally only through access to those activities and facilities that non-disabled people use that disabled people can achieve a role and status that is recognized by society as a whole.

Whilst a person may be able to gain some status within a segregated hospital, hostel or sheltered workplace this is not generally a status that is valued within a wider society. Indeed, the very use of such facilities is often stigmatizing. In order to ameliorate this problem, facilities are given ordinary façades. However, houses in ordinary streets, sheltered workshops on industrial estates and psychiatric wards in general hospitals are all bitter reminders of the way in which people who experience serious ongoing mental health problems have to pretend that they do not if they are to be accepted.

There is a tendency for an exclusive focus on integration to result in a devaluing of relationships between people who are socially disabled. It is normal for people to choose friends and social contacts amongst those with whom they share significant life experiences. For example, most of us have friends who we met at school or college, people who we work with and people with whom we perform leisure activities. Serious mental health problems constitute a significant challenge that can change the whole course of a person's life. It is therefore quite normal for many people who have had this experience to share a common bond. Such bonds can be seen in numerous self-help and segregated social activities that not only offer shelter but, more importantly, offer a place to meet like-minded people. The question clearly arises as to whether such segregated activities and facilities require the input of professionals. Outside the mental health field, amongst other oppressed groups, some forms of segregation are positively valued and called separatism. A degree of separatism has often been important in the struggles of, for example, racial and ethnic minorities as well as lesbians and gays, against the discrimination they experience. The various service user/ex-patient movements and numerous self-help groups and networks, provide a place in which the individual has value not despite but because of their mental health problems. Segregation on service users' own terms, in their own places, can be valuable and constructive. The problems arise when segregation is forced upon someone and takes a form determined by another.

The provision of shelter in some domains can facilitate access to ordinary relationships and activities in others. A few people derive benefit from a sheltered living situation in order to relieve them of some responsibilities so that they can undertake others: social and work roles. Others can live independently and maintain ordinary domestic and family roles if they have some sheltered environment offering support with the maintenance of these roles. The possibilities are many and varied. We know of one women's self-help group that meets just once a week. It provides its members with a place where they can be understood, together with a network of friends who can support each other when difficulties arise: a combination that enables them to sustain ordinary family, domestic and work roles (Good Practices in Mental Health, 1994).

At another level, many people who leave sheltered accommodation and live in the community are extremely isolated. Where insufficient support is available to ensure genuine access to roles and relationships the community can be a very lonely place. Simply because a person is living 'in the community' does not mean that they are a part of it. Where resources do not allow for the necessary level of support to ensure real access, sheltered settings can be valuable in alleviating this social isolation. In addition, there are very few people whose problems and behaviour are unacceptable in the community no matter how much support they have. It is rarely the case that there are no community activities in which such people can partake, but these opportunities may be limited. A sheltered living situation can provide the support a person needs to occupy roles that would otherwise be denied.

It is very important that sheltered settings are reserved for those who really need them. It is often tempting for those managing sheltered facilities, almost unconsciously, to recruit those who are more able. It makes the place easier to run and it is often more satisfying for the staff to see people doing well, but it also deprives those who are more disabled both by removing a place that would otherwise have been available and by fuelling a shift up-market. Standards are set by the more able users and it is not long before those who are more in need of shelter are rejected as too disabled (Sayce *et al.*, 1991). There is also a tendency to fill all places that are available in sheltered accommodation, work and leisure facilities. Disabled people are fitted into these places even if their needs could be met in more ordinary settings.

Finally, although many sheltered environments are also segregated settings this does not have to be the case. Usually we think only about people who are socially disabled using 'ordinary' facilities in the community, but it is equally possible to turn the situation round and think about non-disabled people using sheltered environments designed for those who have mental health problems. This approach has a noble history dating back to early Victorian times when the asylums were major social centres: Charles Dickens attended the Christmas Ball at St Luke's Hospital in 1851 (Showalter, 1987). It is equally possible in many specialist facilities today. Examples in the services in which the present authors work include a sheltered work facility that has a shop-front in an ordinary street and sells its wares to the public, and the renting of rooms and facilities to organizations not connected with mental health services.

Overview: The art of support

The difficulties of people who have serious ongoing mental health problems might best be understood as social disabilities with help and support being directed towards facilitating access to social roles and relationships. In efforts to increase access to social roles and relationships the relationship between those providing support and those requiring assistance is central and critical. Although shelter and support are probably more important in ensuring access than treatment, it is unfortunately the case that within mental health services treatment is often accorded pride of place.

The high status accorded to treatment and therapy and the commensurate devaluing of support and practical help has led to a quite understandable desire for everyone to seek specialist therapeutic skills. We would argue that this is a retrograde step and is likely to detract from the ability of mental health services to facilitate access for those who are socially disabled. Often it is assumed that the provision of support and what has been called 'basic' care is mundane. This is not the case. Providing help and support in a manner that is accessible and acceptable to the people who need it is a sophisticated art. The way in which support and shelter are provided is of the essence if that support is to be effective in assisting the disabled person to develop, grow, gain, retain and use their abilities to the full. Most people who have long term problems have experienced a devaluing serious of failures – with their family, work and friends and then within acute psychiatric services. If support and help imply further failure they can only be destructive.

The provision of support is no simple task: individuals differ, so the meaning of support and the way in which it is provided must be tailored to their needs. To take the supposedly mundane task of helping someone to have a bath as an example. The meaning of being helped to bathe for an individual can vary. We know one older man who enjoyed having someone help him bathe because it made him feel wanted and cared for. For this man, what may be described as 'high-profile' support was most acceptable to him: maximizing the use of bubble bath, helping him to wash his back and allowing him to lie back and soak whilst the staff member chatted to him (and remembered to put in extra hot water when the bath cooled). On the other hand, a younger woman we knew hated help with bathing. Although her physical disabilities and cognitive disorganization made some input necessary, needing help to do something as ordinary as bathe made her feel stupid and useless. In this case a minimalist approach was required: one that made the least fuss, was least obtrusive and made the help as ordinary as possible.

If the support we give is to be positive and non-stigmatizing, the first task is to perform a thorough assessment of the person's wants, wishes, fears, likes, dislikes, values and situation: how do they feel about needing help and how could that help be most acceptably offered? We need actively to move away from the idea that the person should be grateful to us for helping them towards a view that the individual has a right to support and help. The fact that someone is in a position to provide help is a luxury: it affords us a role, status and value that is often denied to the person on the receiving end of our ministrations. This undesirable situation can be altered by changing the values underlying the help.

In services for people who are socially disabled as a consequence of their mental health problems, as with any other services, the helper is there to serve the person who requires assistance. The challenge that this poses will require a great deal of skill and sensitivity: empathy with those in need of support and an overt consideration of how different types of help might feel. Relationships are crucial.

PART TWO

Roles and Relationships

Introduction

The relationship between client and mental health worker is important in all areas, but when working with someone who experiences serious ongoing mental health problems a positive relationship based on honesty and a degree of mutual trust and confidence takes on particular significance. It demands a greater level of skill and sensitivity on the part of the worker. These relationships are at the heart of providing support for people with ongoing mental health problems, and the development and maintenance of relationships constitute the primary component of the specialist skills involved in helping this client group. The success of any endeavour, whether it be assistance with the basics of day to day life, formal therapy, treatment or emotional support, will depend upon the relationship we have with the person we are helping (Repper *et al.*, 1994).

Good relationships do not just 'happen': as Perkins and Dilks (1992) have discussed, neither professional training nor more ordinary experiences equip us for the challenge of working with people whose life experiences and day to day reality are markedly different from our own. Developing an effective relationship with someone who is severely disabled by ongoing mental health problems is a critical and skilled art: one that requires a considerable degree of sensitivity, knowledge and expertise. There is a tendency to blame the social disabilities of clients when relationships go wrong but the responsibility for maintaining relationships lies with the mental health worker. It is not possible for us to succeed or get it right all of the time, but we can recognize when we have gone wrong and learn from our mistakes. Essentially, this process depends above all upon a willingness and ability to learn from the people with whom we work – both the people who are there because they need our support and our colleagues.

In the discussion that follows, we will draw on some of the lessons we and others working in the field have learned. We are not offering a particular formula for successful relationship formation – there can be no such thing. Each and every relationship is different and requires flexibility, adaptation and creativity, a real ability to 'think on one's feet'. Here we hope to offer guidance to fuel this thinking process and some relevant considerations to assist in the delicate process of building effective working relationships.

Chapter 4 draws on research to discuss the general issues involved in forming relationships with people who are seriously disabled. In line with the principles of according clients choice and facilitating the development of their own means of coping, this chapter explores the importance of helping them to come to an understanding of their mental health problems. Chapter 5 offers a more focused consideration of relating to someone whose experience of the world is profoundly different from our own. Specific consideration is given to ways in which we can work with people experiencing acute symptoms and overcome the difficulties posed by cognitive deficits in order to foster positive and progressive relationships. In Chapter 6 some of the common barriers to effective relationship formation are outlined. The importance of supervision is highlighted in the light of the challenges and questions that arise within these relationships.

Creating effective relationships | 4

An 'effective relationship' is not an easy thing to define (Burnard, 1988), especially when working with people severely disabled by ongoing mental health problems. In this context, the effectiveness of the relationship between a client and worker can best be measured by the extent to which the client is facilitated in living the life they wish to live and meeting their own goals. To this end, the relationship needs to provide a safe environment in which the client can consider their own wishes, recognize their own strengths, accept their limitations and mobilize their personal resources. Whilst this might be the purpose of the relationship it is often not fully realized. Workers need to be prepared to spend time fostering mutual trust within the relationship so that the client has the confidence to accept help, or feels sufficiently supported to consider what options are available to them. Every relationship is an individual affair and the possibilities of the alliance will be enhanced or constrained by the attitudes and characteristics of the client and the worker, and the social and situational context in which the relationship is formed.

The characteristics, experiences, beliefs and interests of both client and worker are important in the development of effective relationships. For example, the relationship possibilities and problems between a young, white, newly-qualified graduate nurse and an older, black, working-class mother of three are quite different from those existing between the same nurse and a young man who has just dropped out of college because of his mental health difficulties. In making the most of the possibilities presented by these situations it is essential that opportunities for misunderstandings and resentment that might undermine the development of trust and respect are minimized. In this regard it is helpful to explicitly acknowledge, respect and explore the differences, asking the person about their life, culture, experiences and beliefs, and sharing some of our own. To allow the relationship to develop effectively it is important to carefully consider the meaning of the differences for the client and to use this understanding to inform more sensitive interactions. For example, what will it feel like for an older woman to be told what to do by a nurse who she sees as a 'young girl who knows nothing'? This could be a very demeaning situation, but it can be improved by asking the person what is the best way to do the task in question or minimizing the importance of the help that is given.

A relationship with someone who is compulsorily detained will be quite different from one in which a person is being visited by a staff member in their own home. The former has to juggle the often incompatible demands of a custodial protective role with one which fosters growth, choice and change. The relationship must be able to accommodate and sympathize with all the anger and resentment that the detained person is likely to experience, help them to address some of those factors that lead to the compulsory detention, and at the same time ensure that the conditions of that detention are met. However, in such a situation, the client is generally available to be seen by the staff member – they have to be. This is not the case if a client is living in their own home where they have the right to refuse contact with the mental health worker. In this situation the agenda in relationship formation is a delicate 'wooing' of the client, ensuring that they can see some value in developing the relationship. Whilst they may have many needs that are abundantly clear to the staff worker, these may not be needs that the client defines for him or herself – and it is these latter, self-defined needs that will be important in engaging the client.

An effective relationship with someone who experiences serious ongoing mental health problems is likely to be long lasting and to have a central role in the person's life. In this context issues arise over self-disclosure. As Perkins and Dilks (1992) have argued:

> Some 'self-disclosure', real two way sharing, is essential in forming an effective relationship with someone who has few, if any, other close relationships.

If the person is telling of their life then it is important for the staff worker to tell something of their own, otherwise a two-way interaction cannot occur. Clearly, staff should not engage in painful and sensitive self-disclosures, and the way in which any disclosures may be understood (or misunderstood) by the client must be given careful consideration. Most of us have areas of our life that are safe to share in the process of relationship formation – our views, holidays, cats, interests, leisure and sports pursuits. Telling about ourselves for our own benefit must be avoided, the key question is how will any self-disclosure effect our relationship with the person we are trying to help?

The discovery of common interests can have numerous advantages in the form of demonstrating to the disabled individual that they exist as a person apart from their mental health problems, that they have an expertise or knowledge that is valuable and interesting. In any such discussions it is, of course, vital that the staff member makes a point of listening to the person and giving them an opportunity to air their views however discrepant these may be with their own. It is also important that the worker takes them seriously enough to enter into debate and argument: 'Yes dear, that's an interesting point of view' is a far more demeaning response (and destructive of relationship formation) than is 'I know a lot of people share your views, but I find it difficult to agree'. A balance of valuing the person's opinion and honesty must be struck.

Further to common interests that might be discovered through discussions with clients about their life as a 'person' rather than as a 'patient', such two-way conversations form the basis of a supportive relationship. They reveal a rich and real picture of clients' views of the world, their strengths, ways of coping, patterns of socializing, perceptions of their illness, self-concept and, perhaps most importantly, the way they understand their problems. Strauss (1994) discusses the limitations of traditional psychiatric interviewing and rating scales in gaining a true understanding of clients, and uses case studies to describe the importance of using personal accounts to comprehend clients' perceptions.

Although there is much about relationship formation that is specific to time, person and circumstance, research suggests that some factors are particularly important. Through in-depth interviews with case managers and their clients, Repper *et al.* (1994) identified four main principles of effective working relationships with clients: realism, taking a long term perspective, a positive, empathic, understanding of the client and client-centred flexibility. These principles offer a useful framework to explore further the development of effective relationships with people who experience serious and long term mental problems.

REALISM

Case managers were realistic about progress clients could be expected to achieve. They viewed these limited achievements positively through having an understanding of the client's situation and views.

Repper et al., *1994*

One of the most important characteristics of work with people who have long term problems is realism. In forming effective relationships it is important that the mental health worker is realistic about the very slow (or non-existent) pace of change that might be expected. Much work with people who experience serious ongoing mental health problems is more about enhancing and maintaining their quality of life than improving their clinical or social functioning. However, this maintenance cannot be seen: whereas we can see someone improving (however slowly), we cannot see them failing to get worse. Just as we cannot see insulin maintaining someone who has diabetes, we cannot see a key relationship or supports maintaining someone's work, social network or accommodation in the community – unless, that is, we take it away and the social fabric of their lives breaks down. Accepting the vital role played by maintenance is essential.

However, maintenance is not the only issue, a person's ability to cope might fluctuate: to give an example, a young woman had been admitted at least once a year for the past 10 years. When in hospital she was typically acutely disturbed, disruptive and violent. But, with containment and treatment, she would rapidly improve to a point where, after some 2–3 months, she could return to the supported accommodation where she lived. When well, she was charming – a pleasure for anyone to work with, always vowed never to stop taking her medication again (a factor associated with all relapses) and enthusiastically engaged with the programme that she and her keyworker planned. Over the years, we have heard several keyworkers say 'She is a changed woman now, she's so much better, everything will be all right now, perhaps she could move on to a place of her own soon ...', but it did not last. Invariably, she decided after a few months that she was so well she did not need medication or help and a few months later her ability to cope would deteriorate in a very dramatic way. Then the tone of her keyworkers all too often changed: 'What's the point, she always stops taking her medication, she cannot remain in the community, she needs permanent hospitalization, if she doesn't want to take her medication then there's nothing the service can do to help her ...'

It was when she was unable to cope that this young woman needed the continuity of relationship and confidence of her keyworker. Yet, because of the workers' unrealistic expectations, there was an overwhelming desire to withdraw from her at this stage (as did everyone else she knew). Realism does not mean giving up on a person, but it does mean accepting them for what they are. In this example, more realistic expectations might involve accepting that this woman will (not unreasonably in view of the side-effects and the difficulty coming to terms with relying on drugs) want to stop medication. The mental health worker might try to plan with her what she will do when things start to go wrong and over the years it may be possible to decrease the duration of relapses, their severity and their frequency, and help her to manage them more effectively. Essentially, the keyworker relationship must support people through bad times as well as good and, especially importantly, help to make the most of the good times on the clients' terms, doing the things they want to do, living the life they want to live.

A LONG TERM PERSPECTIVE

Allowing clients and case managers to break goals down into smaller steps, not to rush, to understand setbacks as just part of the 'journey', and to realise that 'what doesn't work today might work tomorrow'.

Repper et al., *1994*

It can be seen from the example above that it is not only realistic expectations but a long term perspective that is crucial in working with someone who experiences serious ongoing mental health problems. In the first instance, it can take a long time to establish a good working relationship. Often, people with serious mental health problems have seen numerous relationships with family, friends and mental health workers break down and disappear. They are often very suspicious of new people and can be understandably reluctant to invest their trust again. Trust and consistency and a plan to support the person on a long term basis are therefore important. As one case manager said:

> I see her twice a week no matter what her mental state or whatever her life is like. She actually finds that difficult at times because her experience in the past has been very different, so when she was well no one has visited and when she's been ill she's had a lot of people, but now she has consistency.

Repper et al., *1994*

Change, when it does come, can be very slow and it is easy to become demoralized and give up. People with serious ongoing mental health problems know more about a long term perspective and the strength and tenacity needed to avoid giving up hope than do many mental health workers. We were talking recently to a woman in her early thirties who had spent all her adult life in hospital in units for people with 'challenging' behaviours. She had a baby, whom she loved very much, but could not care for on her own. Despite enormous improvements in her ability to look after herself, to the point where she was able to leave hospital, the baby was taken into care and adoption proceedings started. We were discussing the long, difficult and distressing period that lay ahead of her – her reply was 'Yes, it's awful, it will be awful, but I'm strong enough to cope. I'll get there in the end. I've always believed I'd get there.'

Over the years change can and does happen (see Harding *et al.*, 1978), and those who have to fight the battles of serious ongoing mental health problems need mental health workers who can stick with them through thick and thin without becoming demoralized and giving up hope. Many people with ongoing mental health problems ask questions like 'What's the point? I've been like this for over a decade?', they do not need the additional burden of staff demoralization at the absence of short term 'success'. Providing a sufficiently long time perspective is taken, vast changes can be seen. We have worked with a smart 30 year old black woman who is now attending college to take her A levels. She spent five years barely surviving in the community when she was able to do little other than lie on her bed, with a worker visiting at least four times a week to do her shopping, cooking, cleaning and making sure that her minimum hygiene requirements were met, and a further five years as a long term psychiatric hospital resident. Another middle-aged man had been resident on numerous acute psychiatric wards, defined as 'difficult' by almost everyone he met, before spending the best part of three years in a rehabilitation unit. Now he has his own place. He does not have a job and requires quite intensive help to keep his flat going, but he enjoys an active social life and has a steady girlfriend. He says that his life is easy now – 'life in hospital was very hard'.

In long term care services, the fact that clients stay around longer than the staff is problematic. Although the notes remain and – if they can be located – provide factual information, they lack the richness of personal memory and cannot provide continuity of relationship. If a long term perspective is to be adopted then staff must have a long term view of working within services. Indeed, working in long term care becomes more interesting the longer one stays because it is only over years that the full richness of clients' lives and the purpose of the service become evident. The odd few months experience is really no experience at all, as it lacks that very long term picture that is the essence of the work with people who experience ongoing difficulties.

Nevertheless, staff will come and go, and it is vital to consider issues of 'handover' not only of responsibility but of relationship. A member of staff who is leaving must recognize the enormous and potentially destructive life event that this will be for a client who has few other relationships, give the person ample warning and help them to work through the loss. A series of joint visits with the new worker, giving them time to benefit from the old relationship and begin to establish a new one is also valuable. Without attention to providing continuity, long term support becomes a series of destructive discontinuities. 'Handover' can be painful for the staff member as it often involves someone they have known for years rejecting them ('I'm glad you're leaving – you were useless anyway'). This is an understandable reaction to the rejection that the loss of a keyworker must mean. Workers should avoid attempts to try to make the client like them again in order to make themselves feel better and understand the rejection for the coping mechanism that it is.

POSITIVE, EMPATHIC UNDERSTANDING OF THE CLIENT

Case managers held a deep conviction that these clients had the same rights as every other individual, and that their strengths and aspirations needed to be positively acknowledged and addressed.

Repper et al., *1994*

One of the most crucial elements in building relationships with anyone – clients, colleagues, friends, lovers, relatives – is an ability and a willingness to understand the life of the other person from where they stand. Although it is never possible to know what life is like for someone else, a preparedness to explore the way the client sees their situation is important (Repper *et al.*, 1994). But it can also be a very difficult thing to do. As we have already seen, the lives and experiences of people who have serious ongoing mental health problems are often profoundly different from those working with them. Mental health workers have rarely experienced the serious cognitive and emotional difficulties of the people they work with; have not experienced the bereavement and losses that these often entail; have not experienced the social disadvantages, discrimination and stigma of being a 'mental patient'; and have not experienced some of the intense and powerful sensations and beliefs that mental health problems can endow.

Often because of these differences of experience, and the demands placed on mental health workers from both within and outside the services in which they work, it is easy to think about clients' behaviour in the terms of the mental health worker. We see someone as being 'difficult' (to us), 'disruptive' (to us), 'non-compliant' (with our prescriptions), 'uncooperative' (with what we are trying to do), 'aggressive' (to us). Whilst these may all be 'true' from where we stand, from where the client stands it often looks very different.

Imagine being a student at college or university, gradually things start to go wrong. You can't think the way you used to. You start to fall behind. People start treating you strangely. You go to the doctor (or are compulsorily taken to the doctor). You are prescribed pills that make you feel bad, tired. But still the problems continue. You get admitted to a hospital where everyone else is 'mad'. You lose your college place. Your friends and your family start treating you differently. No one understands what you are going through. You become a 'mental patient' (with all that this entails) ... and 10 years later you are still there. Are not anger, resentment, frustration and hopelessness very understandable emotions in such circumstances?

If you, as an adult, could not keep your flat in order, could not work, had no friends, imagine the ambivalence you would feel to some mental health worker coming in to help you do things that everyone else could do for themselves: needing help yet not wanting to need it. The anger towards the help provider that this might engender, and the temptation to say 'Go away. I hate you ... I don't need your help ... I never want to see you again ...', whilst at the same time hoping that they will come back anyway because you don't know how you would manage on your own.

An empathic understanding of the client's contradictory feelings about their situation involves a certain humility. 'I know what you mean' is probably one of the most inaccurate and dismissive statements that anyone working with those who experience serious ongoing mental health problems can make. In efforts to understand, it is important to recognize that which we do not understand. There is a huge gulf between a person who is seriously disabled by ongoing mental health problems and a mental health worker who has the job, status, home, friends, family, social life of which their client dreams. Unless one has actually had serious ongoing mental health problems it is not possible to 'know' what life with these difficulties is like. The individual who experiences these problems is the one with this knowledge and if effective relationships are to be formed then this expertise must be both explored and respected. Instead of 'I know what you mean', it might be more accurate to say 'If I were in your place I think I'd feel very angry/frustrated/resentful/hopeless'.

It is only through listening to our clients that we can gain any real insight into what their life is like and we must be willing to learn from them: what different treatments and interventions are like, what is helpful, what is not, what strategies they have developed to cope. A mental health worker who has the privilege of working with numerous clients can in this way accumulate a huge body of knowledge from the expertise of their clients that might be used to help others.

Although we cannot totally empathize with another person's experiences and feelings, we can endeavour to understand their perceptions through careful questioning, observing, discussion and a genuine curiosity. It is vital to want to understand their life, their difficulties, and the impact that the latter has had on the former to produce the person whom one is working with. This is not some form of morbid curiosity – viewing the lunatics at the madhouse – but a genuine desire to explore and relate to people whose lives might be very different from our own (or whose lives might have been quite similar but for serious mental health problems). If we can understand their experiences and their views on life, it helps us to understand what sort of help they want and why they might not want help at all. As one case manager said:

> She feels very strongly on the one hand that she is entitled to services because of what happens to her. On the other hand she does not want to be identified as mentally ill in any way, by her neighbours. It is ambivalence, but it makes sense within the context of her life ... She doesn't want to be involved with me on a day to day basis.

Repper et al., *1994*

In a series of interviews with people with severe social disability, Johnson (1995) explored views of the helpfulness of mental health workers. It was apparent that clients could recognize and articulate the qualities that they valued most in staff. They gave examples of people who were genuinely interested in them, made time to talk to them as another person rather than merely about their mental state, were willing to help them do what they wanted to do (go for a walk, visit the shops, have a bath ...) and shared a sense of humour. In a poignant interview, one client said that once, many years ago, a nurse had given him a bath when he was dirty and 'she talked to me and made me feel warm – nice, as though she hadn't minded doing it all'. Surely we can offer more than this?

The humour that was valued by the clients in the Johnson's study (1995) can be valuable in the formation of any effective relationship. There are often situations where a mental health worker and client can use humour not as a way of minimizing the importance of an event, but as a way of coping with it.

CLIENT-CENTRED FLEXIBILITY

> An individualised approach was crucial, case managers allowed the client
> to set their own agenda and were willing to persevere with a variety of
> strategies over time.
>
> *Repper* et al., *1994*

People who experience serious ongoing mental health problems need help to identify their wishes and mobilize their resources, and being socially disabled they often need help to meet the demands of everyday life. What is more, their needs for support vary over time. The worker therefore has to continuously evaluate what the person needs on this particular occasion and how this can best be provided, treading the thin line between underprovision (or neglect) and overprovision (or deskilling the person), whilst allowing the client to guide the process by prioritizing their needs and wishes. This involves a high level of interpersonal skill and flexibility. Interventions and therapy can rarely be conducted in a formal planned way: instead they must be continually adjusted and tailored around the person's needs. As one case manager said when asked about whether he used 'clinical interventions':

> Yes, the skills I have from other sources like hypnosis, psychotherapy.
> It's not in a planned way, sometimes an opportunity comes up to talk in a
> different way with him. I'll seize that and do it.
>
> Cited in *Repper* et al., *1994*

Formal analytic psychotherapy, or brief focal psychotherapy, are rarely appropriate in building relationships and working effectively with people who have serious mental health problems. However, the skills that these endow may include ways of understanding situations, the range of possible responses or courses of action, and the implications of each of these. It could be argued that 'clinical interventions' with such clients involve an extremely sophisticated use of psychotherapeutic skills, as well as day to day personal support skills. But these have to be tailored to the individual's specific needs and problems at a particular moment in time. If effective relationships are to be fostered, 'fitting in' with how the client feels is important. The mental state of one man we knew fluctuated a great deal. Every time we called it was necessary to perform a very rapid assessment. On days when his 'voices' were troubling him he liked to simply sit for a few moments and talk about the weather: a visit longer than five minutes exacerbated his difficulties, as did any more intense conversation. At such times he had problems with looking after himself, so we helped him with any essential sorting out of his flat and shopping without asking him to help and often in silence. On other days, he would be more able to welcome us. These were days for a practical, problem-solving approach very much in the 'here and now'. He would raise difficulties and we would explore the options available to him, as well as jointly doing any necessary practical tasks. At a third level, there were times when he was not overwhelmed by his symptoms, but thoughtful about them. At these times, it was possible to discuss some of the therapeutic approaches to deal with hearing voices and unusual beliefs and work out how he might utilize these. Finally, there were times when he wanted to focus on his life and the many bereavements he had suffered (loss of his wife, job, home) as a consequence of his mental health problems. Here approaches and understandings from bereavement counselling were appropriate.

The working relationship with this client involved a series of different approaches – practical help, emotional support, problem-solving techniques, specific symptomatic interventions and bereavement work carried out simultaneously, but not in a continuous fashion. It might, for example, be several weeks between one 'bereavement' discussion and the next. Therefore, it was important for the mental health worker to carry these different strands across long periods of time.

At a more straightforward level, flexibility in frequency, duration and location of contact are important. Sometimes a client wants to talk for a protracted period of time, at others a brief contact is all that is needed/possible and pressing on regardless is positively destructive. At some times a client needs only infrequent visits, but at others may value daily contact. Similarly, some people, at some times, prefer someone to visit them, at others they want to get out of their home. In order to maintain contact and to build a trusting relationship it is essential that clients are not always expected to attend pre-set appointments in a mental health service. Although this may be appropriate, and might be agreed between client and worker, some people will prefer to meet at teatime in a local café. For others a relationship might need to be built up around 'chance' meetings, opportunities to check they are okay, to offer further support if it is necessary and to demonstrate a consistent and long term interest and concern.

Most importantly, as far as possible, clients should have control over the help they receive. The possibility of seeing someone when they feel the need to do so is just as important to someone who experiences serious ongoing mental health problems as it is to the rest of the population. There are many ways in which this can be achieved. One woman lived in a flat and most of the time liked to manage her life by herself with a mental health worker calling round for a chat on a weekly basis. However, there were times when her 'ideas' got worse (and in the past she had made numerous suicide attempts). In recognition of this need, she was given a variety of 'points of contact' with people she knew so that she could avail herself of the help she needed at any particular time.

It is most useful if the receipt of help and support is determined by the client him/herself rather than the service provider. Although there are obviously constraints in terms of available resources and expertise, it is important not only to have a range of things to offer, but wherever possible to allow the client to be in control of what they receive.

USER'S CHOICE

Most mental health strategy documents pay lip-service to the importance of responding to users' views and wishes – to giving users choice. If this is to be any more than empty rhetoric then it is vital that as providers we accept the wishes of people with mental health problems wherever possible, even if they are at odds with our own opinions. We cannot expect clients to begin to trust us unless we can demonstrate that we trust them by responding to and acceding to their views, we may explain our reservations about their opinions but the ultimate choice is theirs. Clearly, there are times when the law requires that we override the client's judgement, but there are many other ways in which we deny the individual's right to choose. In particular, we fail to make them aware of the range of options available; fail to help them pursue their chosen course of action when it differs from what we think best; and make one form of help or support contingent upon another.

Unless any of us is aware of the options available, we cannot consider the pros and cons of each and make a decision about which would suit us best. No one has a completely unconstrained choice – the choices available to all of us are determined by the personal, social and material resources available. We do not have a free choice about where we live – it is constrained first by finances, then by proximity to our work, and/or our partners work, and/or our children's schools, and/or its capacity to house all those with whom we want to live, not to mention our DIY and gardening abilities if work is required on the property. Similarly, our choices about work are constrained by our qualifications and experience and ability to acquire these, our interests, geographical restrictions, the money we need to earn to support other obligations we have and, most importantly, those jobs that are available in the local labour market.

Although our choices about what we want to do with our lives are constrained by circumstances, they are not absent, but in order to exercise that choice we need to know two things: what the limits on our choices are and what each of the available choices would be like. Sometimes staff modify the truth by selecting the information they make available to clients. For example, in hospitals designated for closure we have seen numerous instances of residents being asked where they want to live and replying that they want to stay where they are which is, of course, impossible. The person experiences having their opinions ignored when they are eventually forced to move in order to facilitate closure. To be offered choice and then ignored is more damaging than not having a choice: the person receives the message that their views are not worth listening to and the relationship between client and worker is damaged. Most of us would be unlikely to trust someone who asked us what we wanted and then did something completely different. We would be unlikely to bother offering our opinions again. What would be the point?

If people are to have real choices then honesty is important. Workers must explain that the hospital will close, outline the real choices that are actually available and sympathize with the understandable anger when what the person really wants is not possible. It is only when the person knows what is available in terms of geographical location, proximity to facilities and services, and type that they are able to make a real choice.

We also deny a person choice when we only tell them about one option, or when we only allow them access to limited information about the other choices. In effect, we make the choice for them and only tell them about the conclusion we have reached. Unless a person has information about the range of choices – for example, what it is like taking haloperidol rather than chlorpromazine, having ECT rather than taking antidepressant medication or having cognitive therapy – then choice is meaningless. For a person to choose the options available we can give them detailed verbal descriptions, or we might give the person the opportunity to try the different options, or we could arrange for them to meet people who have tried the different alternatives.

One of the most common ways of denying a person choice involves the withdrawal, or failure to provide, support and help when a person makes a choice that does not accord with the option selected by the worker. Choice is only meaningful if the person is allowed to make 'wrong' choices and receive support in pursuing them. We deny choice when, for example, we tell someone they are free to leave a hostel or hospital that they do not like without helping them to find alternative accommodation and providing support there, or when we say they are welcome to go and look for a job but fail to provide them with help to find, get and sustain work.

In a more overt way, we often deny choice when we only allow a person access to a service that they want if they agree to take up a further type of help that we think they should receive: make one form of help contingent upon another. For example, it is not uncommon for a person only to be allowed lunch at a day centre if they go to a group first, only have a CPN visit if they take their medication. This type of approach is dangerous: it not only denies choice but often excludes the person from any help at all. It is destructive to any relationship between services and the client.

One way in which clients can gain some control of their situation is through an understanding of their problems: if they are unaware of why they feel the way they do, what might make their life so much more difficult and so different from that of others, they can feel helpless and, not infrequently, hopeless. Clients need information about the different ways in which they can make sense of their experiences. Too often workers only describe their own chosen theories and deny access to those of others. Choice applies equally to styles of life and ways of understanding problems.

THEORIES, UNDERSTANDINGS AND EXPLANATIONS OF DISABILITY

Everyone seeks explanations for what is going on in the world and what is happening to them. Some of the time we approach health services for help because we want to know what is wrong with us and what can be done about it.

However, some explanations will make more sense to us than others: we need an explanation that we can understand in terms of the way in which we view the world. At other times we believe we know what is wrong with us, we have already constructed our own explanations (which may or may not accord with those of the professional we consult) and want the help indicated by our chosen explanations. We are often very reluctant to accept any treatment that is not consistent with our views about what is wrong with us. The models we hold determine our attitudes towards help and our health related behaviour (Leventhal *et al.*, 1980). Literature on coping (see Lazarus and Folkman, 1984) confirms that the way in which we appraise the meaning of an event determines the coping strategies we use. The theories that anyone holds are important and people with serious ongoing mental health problems are no different.

Within the mental health field there are an ever increasing number of theories about mental health difficulties, all of which can provide supporting evidence for their claims but on none of which a judicious man or woman would bet their life savings! Mainstream professionals have developed numerous biomedical, psychological and social explanations of mental distress (see Siegler and Osmond, 1976). The relative lack of success of these in providing the much sought after 'cures' has no doubt fuelled the growing number of 'alternative' theories which invoke spiritual, religious and nutritional concepts together with ideas from other (mainly eastern) medical systems (see Podvoll, 1992).

Many people with serious ongoing mental health problems initially seek a label for their distress – a diagnosis. It has been considered detrimental to 'label' people as this has been suggested to result in self-fulfilling behaviour on the part of the individual, and to influence their psychiatric management and social treatment (see Scheff, 1967). This approach continues in some places to the present time, but rather than no label being attached to the individual, professionals generally decide upon a diagnosis – which underlies much of the subsequent treatment – but withhold this diagnosis from the client. Although this reluctance is based on the supposed destructive consequences of labelling someone as mad, in itself it can be destructive in the building of any trust with the individual – who is essentially being deceived by those 'caring' for him/her. It is also insulting in that it implies that the individual cannot cope with being told their diagnosis, when many people actually seek a label for their distress. It also precludes any opportunity for the individual to understand what staff in mental health services are doing and why they are doing it.

Furthermore, arguments against labelling people as 'mentally ill' often represent stark naïvety on the part of the mental health professionals. First, it is difficult to see how someone who has serious ongoing mental health problems, is in and out of psychiatric hospital or living in a 'mental health hostel' is not already labelled as 'mad' by the public at large. The absence of diagnosis does not change this popular construction. Second, they imply that there is nothing worse than being labelled 'mad'. Many other oppressed groups – lesbians, gays, people with Aids – have actively adopted the oppressive labels applied to them and used these as the basis for fighting their oppression. Similar moves can be seen in the mental health user movement with the adoption of the label 'mad' in a similar political manner.

People may accept or reject the label that we as professionals think is correct, but in order to do so they must know what it is and what it means. It is worth also being aware of some of the controversies over whether 'schizophrenia' or 'personality disorder' actually exist (Johnstone, 1989; Bentall *et al.*, 1988; Boyle, 1990). It is sometimes useful to discuss these debates with clients, but it is never enough to stop at a label. The next step is to consider what that label means. Here a basic knowledge of the range of outcomes of serious mental health problems (see Ciompi, 1988; Harding *et al.*, 1978), together with the theories or models used for understanding the person, are vital. When clients ask 'What is happening/has happened to me?' or 'What is wrong with me?' they deserve answers.

There is no one 'correct' theory about mental health problems. Therefore, it is vital that professionals have some understanding of at least the major medical, psychological and social theories that have been put forward (see Siegler and Osmond, 1976), together with an awareness of the models employed in cultures other than their own from which their clients might come (see Helman, 1984). When deciding which model might be most appropriate in helping a person to understand their difficulties, there are at least three important considerations: first the model must make an explicit link between the supposed 'underlying' problems and the client's experiences; second, it must make sense to the client. There are no 'proven facts' about what causes serious ongoing mental health problems, there are merely a lot of theories. Science cannot therefore be the arbiter but the theories must be meaningful to the people who have to live with the difficulties. Third, it must have heuristic value. That is, it must help the client to move closer to living the life they wish to live, and it must help both client and the worker to generate ideas, approaches and interventions that are useful in assisting the person to reach his or her goals.

Often, different models are quite compatible with each other but provide different types of explanations. For example, it is possible to believe that neurotransmitter systems become faulty (medical model), that this influences the person's ability to control the contents of consciousness (cognitive/psychological model) and that both of these events can be precipitated by traumatic life events such as child sexual abuse (psychoanalytic model) and/or disrupted social relationships and social disadvantages (social model).

Neither does a single model imply a particular approach to treatment. Medication, for example, may be construed as treating the 'root cause' of the person's problems or as helping to ameliorate the influence of destructive social circumstances or psychological damage wrought in early childhood. As with any other intervention, there does not have to be a reflexive relationship between treatment and cure. In much the same way as aspirin alleviates headaches, but headaches are not caused by aspirin deficit, so drugs, and environmental, social and psychological interventions may alleviate the consequences of serious mental health problems even if none of these are causal of the person's problems.

The critical issues in helping a person to understand their situation revolve around whether a theory makes sense to the person and whether it helps them get where they are trying to go. Some people have already adopted 'standard' explanations for their problems: 'It's all because of my brain', 'It's all because of my family'. If this is the case, then it is worth while exploring a little more what this means to the person: there are some people for whom there is a rider to such comments, '... therefore I am hopeless and useless and there is nothing I can do'. These people have no sense of their own ability to take control of their situation and a gentle reframing of their understanding that endows a greater sense of agency and optimism, whilst acknowledging the very real difficulties faced, might be useful: 'the things that are wrong with your brain/family do not mean that you cannot do anything. Your problems may make these things harder, but not impossible.' It is sometimes useful to give examples of other people with similar problems who work and have their own homes, but care must be taken not to make the individual feel they have failed in the light of others' achievements.

Some people have adopted 'non-standard' explanations for their problems. When this occurs, professionals often declare the person to lack insight and attempt to alter their beliefs (see Perkins and Moodley, 1993b). This may not be desirable or useful and implies a certain arrogance on the part of mental health workers: insight, after all, basically means agreeing with the professional (David, 1990). It is entirely possible that the person's own explanation makes sense to them and is useful in allowing them to adopt strategies that enable them to live the life they choose. For example, one woman believed that her problems resulted from having offended God by spending her time with friends, drinking, having sex and so on as a child rather than going to church. She wanted to get back to being a good Christian and so tried extremely hard to attend all church services and events (even though this was difficult for her on occasions) and was delighted with the progress she was making. She would accept all help designed to assist her towards this end, including medication (to help her organize her thoughts enough to pray properly), practical support and reading classes (to enable her to read the Bible and other texts). There was little to be gained from trying to change her beliefs and, potentially, much to be lost.

On other occasions, non-standard theories may require some modification, but it is important that workers are sensitive to the types of model with which the client is most comfortable. For example, one young man with serious ongoing mental health problems believed he had something wrong with the nerves in his chest and that this was likely to give him a heart attack. This meant that at the age of 22 years he had effectively taken to his bed – he would take psychotropic medication but do little else. Clearly, this man liked physical explanations and we decided to agree that he had trouble with his nerves, but those in his head rather than in his chest. In conjunction with the necessary medical tests to check that his heart was sound, diagrams of neurotransmitters and the way nerve cells operate were used to suggest alternative constructions. Such explanations allowed him to understand why he may have had difficulty in going out and to begin to work out ways of doing some of the things he used to enjoy like meeting friends and going to the pub. Such a process may be protracted but it is always important to use those things that the person wants to be able to do, rather than those which they 'ought' to do, in order to facilitate it. It is likely that this young man would still be in bed if initial efforts had been directed towards cleaning his room.

Similar considerations apply if a person does not have any well constructed theories or explanations for their problems. The clinician must be sensitive to the way in which the client describes other aspects of their world, and offer choices. Often it is useful to say 'Well there are a lot of different theories ...' and briefly, at a level appropriate to this person's educational background, go through a medical, a social and a psychological theory, trying to identify the ways in which each might be relevant to the person's experience. Often, when something is said that strikes a chord, the person will chip in with an example from their own life. Literature produced by such organizations as MIND and the NSF can be helpful in this process. On other occasions individually tailored materials may be more useful.

Theories and models of mental health difficulties may seem a long way from issues relating to the formation of effective worker/client relationships. In fact they are central to this process First, unless client and mental health worker can reach a shared understanding of the person's difficulties it is unlikely that the worker will be able to offer the support that is acceptable to the client and present it in an appropriate manner. Second, the model adopted is critical in determining the view of both client and worker concerning the possibilities open to the individual and the things they might do in life.

It is also the case that too little time has been spent talking to people who experience serious mental health problems about the nature of their problems and possible solutions: users frequently complain about being given too little information (Sandford, 1994). The opportunity to discuss mental health problems, both in general and specific terms, is greatly valued by many people and is an essential part of developing effective relationships. Such discussions can be an important part of a more general counselling process helping the person to live with the losses that their problems have entailed (work, friends, family, the life they had expected to live) and adapt to a life that includes mental health difficulties.

Approaches and difficulties | 5

The cognitive and emotional difficulties experienced by people who have serious mental health problems can impede access to roles and relationships. It is therefore important to consider how their disabling effects can be minimized (Hatfield, 1989; Perkins and Dilks, 1992). How 'should' we respond to strange and unusual ideas and experiences? How can we overcome the difficulties posed to relationships by cognitive confusion, poor concentration and attentional deficits?

In this chapter we will focus on the relationship between client and mental health worker, but all of the issues considered are equally applicable to other relationships. They can be used by mental health workers in facilitating interactions between the client and families, friends, neighbours and colleagues. However, it must again be stressed that there can be no 'cookery-book' formula for working with individuals' problems. Instead, it is important that the mental health worker understands the principles and issues involved and applies these in a flexible manner that is appropriate for the particular person with whom they are working.

STRANGE AND UNUSUAL BELIEFS

Probably one of the most unhelpful myths that pervades most mental health work is that 'you must never collude with a delusion'. If a person expresses a delusional idea then it should be ignored, diverted or challenged (for example, Watts *et al.*, 1973). The origins and validity of this belief are not wholly clear, yet it is certainly widely held, and at first sight seems intuitively sensible. If a person says something that is manifestly 'untrue' (in the eyes of the professional and everyone else) then they should be encouraged to see the error of their ways. However, as mental health workers it is important to move beyond the intuitive and examine the implications and consequences of such an approach.

First, a belief that one must challenge and divert delusional beliefs does not accord with the definition of a delusion as a fixed, false belief, i.e. not susceptible to confirmation or disconfirmation by external events. If this is the case, what is the point of challenging delusions? A person who holds strange and unusual beliefs will have had these beliefs challenged or ignored by just about everyone they meet ('Don't be silly', 'That's rubbish', 'Yes dear, would you like a cup of tea?') and still they hold that belief. Why should someone else challenging them be any more effective?

Second, it is not only the case that challenging or ignoring a person's unusual beliefs is unlikely to be effective in changing them: such a strategy usually actively mitigates against effective relationship formation. It renders them further isolated and alone:

> To deny another's reality, to ignore and divert what may be very frightening experiences, serves to further isolate them and effectively prevents the formation of a good working relationship. If you knew that you would be arrested if you went outside your house you would expect someone trying to help you to appreciate, empathise with, and understand, your distress, not ignore or avoid it.

Perkins and Dilks, 1992

In forming a relationship with someone who has ideas that seem strange and unusual to others four principles are important:

1. **Avoid trivializing or disregarding delusions.** However bizarre the person's ideas may seem to others, they are real for that person. There is a temptation to disregard unusual beliefs as if they cannot really be true. This is a mistake, they are very real for the person concerned. A belief that one is about to be poisoned, receives special messages from the newscaster on the television or is the Virgin Mary, is just as real for that person as our beliefs that we are a clinical psychologist and a research fellow. If someone denies or trivializes things that are important to us, that we know to be true, then this actively mitigates against us forming a relationship with them.

2. **Take cultural factors into account.** In understanding a person's beliefs, it is important to accept that everyone's reality is different. The myriad belief systems that prevail in the world, and within any one culture, are ample demonstration that there is not an absolute external 'reality'. We, as children of a modern western culture, are steeped in a belief system where objectivity and 'science' predominate. This is entirely alien to one whose understanding of the world embodies ideas about spirits, deities and supernatural powers that are equally implausible to us. Within our own culture, ideas about intrapsychic processes – ids, egos, superegos, inner children and cognitive schemata – are treated as 'facts' by those who believe in them, and as ridiculous inventions by those who do not (see Kitzinger and Perkins, 1993). Our

understanding of events and experiences is quite different depending upon our belief system and the values we hold: a wolf-whistle will be understood as a form of flattery by some readers of this book and as offensive 'sexual harassment' by others.

The belief systems of our clients, however strange and unusual, can be understood in this framework: another way of understanding reality. There is, however, an important difference in that their beliefs are typically shared by no one else. Although there are important precedents for this (the status of Jesus Christ was, we believe, denied by many at the time) most people can find others who share their beliefs. The absence of such kindred spirits renders the individual alone in a struggle of trying to balance the demands of the world that those around them experience with their own internal reality. This is a battle in which the person needs allies – and the relationship with a mental health worker who tries to understand their situation can be invaluable.

3. **Explore the implications of the beliefs.** Even if a person is alone in their beliefs, the fact that they hold these beliefs so strongly means that their behaviour is frequently determined by them. Someone who knows they are about to be poisoned will not eat the poisoned food and may well become angry (even violent) towards the presumed poisoner. The beliefs, however strange, constitute the person's world. If we want to know that person, to relate to them, then we must explore their world. We must explore not only that part of their world that makes sense to us (their history, family, friends, circumstances) but also that part which may not (their beliefs, ideas, perceptions). It is only by doing this that we can form an effective working relationship and help them to explore the possibilities that may be open to them.

This does not mean that all behaviour that is a consequence of their belief system will be acceptable to us. There are, for example, some practices within one belief system that are unacceptable – banned – within others: Moslems cannot drink alcohol in some Arab states. Nevertheless, in order to know what a person might do that is unacceptable to others, one has to understand their belief system and accept it as being real for them.

4. **Respond flexibly.** Although a person's beliefs constitute their reality, any belief may be more or less firmly held. There are some beliefs that are core to our understanding of the world and others about which we are less sure, that we check out. There is considerable evidence that strange and unusual ideas vary both from individual to individual and within any one individual across time and circumstances (Brett-Jones *et al.*, 1987). Such variations can be important in tailoring approaches to the individual and, as discussed above, responding flexibly to the client's needs at different times.

There are numerous strategies that mental health workers might adopt in forming relationships with someone who experiences strange and unusual beliefs and it is likely that within any one client/mental health worker relationship all will be appropriate in some situations at some times. Whilst it is important to take a person's beliefs seriously, it is also important never to lie. Dishonesty is destructive of any relationship. There can be a fine line between acknowledging another's reality that is discrepant from one's own and dishonesty – saying that you, yourself, agree with this reality.

It is often the case that someone is unsure about what is happening: 'Is everyone laughing at me?', 'Are they poisoning the food?' The person is trying desperately to cling on to the reality that others share, but which is only tenuously within their grasp (Perkins and Dilks, 1992). In such situations reassurance is a vital life line. Sometimes people are reluctant to provide it because they see the person as 'attention seeking' and being 'a nuisance'. The individual in such circumstances may be seeking attention, but they need attention: help to work out what is going on. Such reassurance may be needed repeatedly and this can be a nuisance, but it is often vital to the person concerned. Some people will be able to acquire the skills of reassuring themselves – working out alternative explanations of what might be going on, following the model set by a mental health worker. Others will require the 'reality check' of reassurance indefinitely.

Sometimes, especially if the person is particularly distressed, simple, clear reassurance is appropriate: 'No they're not laughing at you/trying to poison you'. At other times, if the person is able to consider what is happening at greater length, they may be able to think through alternative explanations themselves: 'Can you think of any other reasons why they might be laughing?' If a person repeatedly requires reassurance at times when the mental health worker is not present then other strategies might be possible. One woman we knew frequently believed that her fire alarm was a bug – especially at night in her flat when no one else was there. A simple note near the gadget saying 'I'm not a bug, just a fire alarm here to protect you' was very helpful.

If a person's unusual beliefs are more firmly held then reassurance that they are not true is no reassurance at all: the person simply becomes frustrated at being unable to convince those who are supposed to be helping them of what they know to be happening. In such a situation one useful approach is to attempt to put oneself in the situation of believing what the client believes and empathize with the emotional impact of that belief rather than its factual content. One young man was extremely distressed because he knew that everyone in his hostel was laughing and talking about him. The mental health worker's response of taking his distress seriously with comments like 'That must feel awful', 'I think that would make me feel that there was something odd about me', 'That must make it very difficult to be around the others' provided at least some of the reassurance he needed. It avoided either denying his reality or being dishonest and agreeing with his construction of events. Listening, sympathizing and empathizing can go a long way.

There are occasions when a person's unusual belief, whilst not real in the experience of others, conveys an emotional quality quite accurately. Whilst it may not have been 'true' that everyone was talking about, and laughing at, the young man described above, it is entirely possible that he felt different and apart from others: this was his way of understanding how he felt. Alternatively, if he looked 'odd' or 'mad' to others, he may have had a great deal of experience of people looking at him and laughing at him and may be particularly sensitive to this. Everyone who has worked in this field must have experienced going out with some clients and being given a wide berth on the footpath, having people move away in pubs, on buses, in shops. These are very real, although rarely acknowledged, horrors with which it is relatively easy to empathize.

Because they are so often disbelieved, it is not infrequent for a client to tell a mental health worker of their beliefs and to seek reassurance that they are believed: 'They're all talking about me, you do believe me don't you?' In such a case it is rarely appropriate to say either 'yes' or 'no': 'yes' is dishonest, 'no' denies the individual's reality. A more useful way of approaching the situation is to move away from the belief that there is any absolute or fixed way of under-standing what is going on in the world. A response to the effect of 'I believe that what you are saying is true for you, but I have no evidence of it'; 'Everyone has a different understanding of reality – what is true for one person is not true for another', 'Perhaps you could tell me a bit more about it' allows the mental health worker to take seriously the individual's reality, empathize with it and explore it further. It also offers the individual a way of understanding why other people may deny their beliefs: understandings which can be helpful in allowing them to cope with other situations. Any situation will be understood differently by the different people involved whether or not these people have mental health problems.

Although a person's strange and unusual beliefs may be very firmly held it is sometimes the case that within them changes are possible. This type of approach probably comes closest to 'colluding with a delusion', but it can be used to good effect in minimizing the destructive consequences of a belief system that is not shared by others. A thorough exploration of a belief system often reveals that particular problematic behaviours do not automatically follow from the beliefs held. One man was absolutely convinced (despite reassurances from the police to the contrary) that he had committed a motoring offence 10 years previously and was continuously ringing the local police station at great length to confess to these. Not only was this causing irritation at the police station, it was also build-ing a telephone bill that was becoming beyond his capacity to pay. It also rendered him unable to do anything until he was arrested. Over a period of time, although his beliefs remained fixed, they were modified in two ways. First, we suggested to him, with much supporting evidence, that when the police want someone they are quick enough to go round and get them so there was really no need to keep ringing to confess. Second, that if he were to be arrested, it might be a good idea to make the most of his remaining freedom and do all the things he wanted to. He was soon seeing friends and going to the pub – with his hood pulled up to reduce the possibility of recognition.

An understanding of a person's belief systems can be important in working out ways of minimizing its disrupting effect on a person's life. First, it may be possible to allow a person to act on their beliefs in a limited way that is not disruptive but does reduce their frustration. One man with whom we worked believed that he was the 'second coming'. He believed it was his mission to preach this truth and he had been excluded from numerous community facilities (bingo halls, social clubs, shops, etc.) where handing out gospel tracts and preaching was considered disruptive. Helping him to become engaged with a local evangelist movement, go to Bible classes and hand out leaflets in places where it would be less disruptive (the London Underground was just fine, and he had a travel pass!) enabled him to pursue his mission and develop links in the community, whilst at the same time reducing the disruption and consequent complaints.

Second, there are occasions when fairly ordinary behaviours can be particularly distressing for an individual because of their significance within their belief system. One man believed that he was dead. This did not interfere with his day to day life unless he was asked 'How are you?' He then described in detail how he had died, how he was being kept alive, and became extremely distressed and unable to do anything for a number of hours. The simple strategy of avoiding a common phrase made an enormous difference.

Third, an understanding of a person's delusional system can indicate where practical supports may be necessary. One woman who believed that her nose controlled the weather was generally able to look after herself. However, when the sun shone she could not go out because she knew that she would make it rain. At such times she was unable to get her shopping and needed someone else to do it for her if she was to continue to live in her own home.

Fourth, even if no changes can be made, an understanding of a person's belief system can warn of problems. A man who believed that people were trying to kill him would gradually come to know that a particular person had murderous intent. Although he would try to restrain himself, when the knowledge became irresistible he simply had to act on it. Although his violence was unprovoked it was predictable because he was able to tell staff when he believed that someone was going to kill him and they could then prevent the violence occurring (usually by offering both parties protection by ensuring they were in different areas).

People who experience serious ongoing mental health problems are particularly vulnerable to stressful events, particularly social events, that most people take within their stride. The anxiety that such events engender can exacerbate a person's difficulties (Brown and Birley, 1968; Day *et al.*, 1987; Ambelas, 1979, 1987; Falloon *et al.*, 1984). It is not just major life events that have a deleterious effect. In a particularly vulnerable individual, simply talking to someone, or being with a group of people, can be more than they can tolerate. This vulnerability to social stressors has implications for relationship formation. At a very basic level, the length of interactions must be sensitively adjusted to that which a person can handle: overlong conversations with the mental health worker can be positively deleterious. One of us has a client who can rarely tolerate interactions of more than 15 minutes before she becomes visibly distressed and her unusual ideas more prominent. Another young man has to take 'cigarette' and 'tea' breaks several times during a session (Perkins and Dilks, 1992) – over the years these breaks have decreased in number.

Such problems can make the mental health worker feel as if they are 'doing nothing', but this is often not the case. For example, one client looked forward to meeting his keyworker each week: he was out waiting for her arrival every time, always offered her a cup of tea, kept his appointment card carefully and insisted that a new appointment was written down each time. He was also well able to dictate how long the keyworker stayed: and it was rarely long enough for her to get more than a couple of sips of her tea. When he had as much contact as he could tolerate he got out his appointment card, ensured a new date was written down and showed her to the door. A half-hour journey for what rarely exceeded a five minute interaction may seem something of an imbalance, but its importance was revealed when the keyworker was off sick. The client became very distressed, phoned the mental health team almost daily reporting numerous physical and social difficulties, and admission was only averted by another worker performing the five minute weekly visits.

Sometimes, doing something with a person can be less distressing than direct conversation where all attention focuses on the individual concerned. A weekly swimming session with the non-threatening snatches of conversation that this allows may be a much more fertile basis for both relationship formation and interventions than a formal 'session'.

Because people with ongoing mental health problems are often socially isolated, there is a temptation to exhort them to 'socialize'. This may be appropriate for some but it can also be positively toxic. Many people have learned through years of experience how to titrate the amount of social stimulation they receive and withdraw when it is at a level that they cannot tolerate – this knowledge should be respected. It may involve the person withdrawing from activities, sitting alone in their accommodation or sitting on the edge of a group but not participating: exhortations to 'join in' may be destructive, increasing stress/anxiety and thereby troubling symptoms. Instead, it may be far more important to allow the person to do as much as they can without unnecessary pressure and ensure that they have things to do that do not necessitate potentially damaging levels of social contact. For example, one severely disabled young man has a thriving car-washing business facilitated by his keyworker who performs some of the interactions with customers which he finds difficult.

COGNITIVE CONFUSION

Many socially disabled people experience a profound confusion, thought disorder and attention/concentration problems. All of these can be an enormous source of distress and severely impede relationship formation. Often the internal world of a person with serious ongoing mental health problems is extremely disorganized – and this can be terrifying (Hatfield, 1989). Most people have had brief glimpses of how frightening it is not to know what is going on, but when this becomes a frequent occurrence, and is combined with an inability to organize and hold on to one's thoughts, the terror that ensues can be great. Unfortunately, it is not possible to see that a person's thoughts are confused and the confusion itself makes it difficult for the person to describe what they are experiencing and can leave the mental health worker feeling unable to cope.

> Statements such as 'I don't know what's going on – do you know what's going on?', 'Please help me – save me please' can be extremely difficult when the person cannot articulate from what they need to be saved or what it is that they do not understand, but simply experience an overwhelming, confusing sense of foreboding.

Perkins and Dilks, 1992

Probably the first step in helping a person who experiences cognitive confusion is to have a way of understanding their difficulties. This is particularly important because part of the individual's fear results from a failure to understand what is going on – a failure that is common to most other people they meet. There are probably many models that could be employed by the worker and we do not intend to arbitrate between these here. However, we have found that the various 'cognitive overload' models (Frith, 1979; Hemsley, 1987) make sense to many clients, and are helpful in generating ways of intervening and circumventing some of the difficulties experienced.

These models basically argue that a person is unable to filter out irrelevant information from the outside world or to limit the contents of consciousness. They are therefore in a state of 'cognitive overload' with too much going on in their head at any one time and unable to focus on any one part of it: their internal world is, therefore, confused and disorganized. These difficulties in the process of thinking cause problems in the performance of even apparently simple tasks. Basic tasks like getting up in the morning involve a large cognitive component (deciding what time to get up, setting the alarm clock, getting out of bed when the alarm clock rings, deciding what to wear, which elements of personal hygiene have to be attended to and in what order). Planning what to do, monitoring it, doing it, modifying what to do if circumstances change ... these are essential cognitive components of all tasks. If one is experiencing serious cognitive confusion then all activities of life become difficult if not impossible. This is poignantly demonstrated by Strauss (1994) who describes the way that one woman marked her recovery by her ability to decide that she wanted the radio on, then follow this through by switching on the radio and subsequently choosing the music that she wanted to hear. The complexity of such a sequence of thoughts and behaviours is rarely considered by those of us for whom these activities are almost automatic.

Cognitive confusion, combined with altered perceptions and strange and unusual ideas, also result in attention and concentration problems. If a person is having difficulty in organizing their thoughts then it is doubly difficult to organize themselves in relation to the external world. It is all too easy to become distracted from what you are doing by both internal and external events. Attention and concentration difficulties can seriously impede even the most basic tasks: one man we knew repeatedly let his bath overflow (much to the consternation of his neighbours). Even simple behaviours like boiling a kettle, and pleasures like writing, reading and meditating, become extremely difficult in the presence of attention and concentration problems: other activities, like smoking a cigarette or cooking, can be positively dangerous.

Further, attention and concentration problems often make a person appear, to others, unreliable, lazy and uncommitted and can therefore seriously jeopardize relationships. If a person does not do what they say they will do, fails to keep appointments, is not there when you call, then this readily engenders frustration and anger. Not only does such behaviour often lead to exclusion from ordinary activities, it can also lead mental health workers to get fed up and withdraw: 'What's the point, he's never there, he can't be bothered'. This is a mistake. The person is excluded from services because of the very problems that render them in need of those services. Cognitive confusion, attention and concentration difficulties are part of what characterizes serious ongoing mental health problems, and therefore the relationships that we build and the services we provide must accommodate them. If this is not the case then it is rather like denying a person a wheelchair because they are unable to walk to get it.

Difficulties in thinking should not be confused with lack of intellect. A person who has difficulties in the process of thinking is no more likely to be stupid or clever than anyone else, but their ability to use their assets to their full potential may be affected. However, like strange and unusual ideas, cognitive confusion, attention and concentration difficulties are not stable over time. A person who is unable to tolerate any interaction on one occasion may be well able to converse at length on another, necessitating a considerable degree of flexibility on the part of the mental health worker. It is also possible to capitalize on this variability and ensure that the individual has the opportunities to use their abilities to the full at those times when they are most capable of doing so.

If a person is experiencing cognitive confusion they have difficulty in organizing their internal world. As this causes problems in organizing their external world then one way of helping them is to provide the external structure that they are unable to provide for themselves. In this context several things can be useful: diaries, timetables, prompts, reminders and regular routines. The availability of work can be particularly important in this regard. Some people will, quite naturally, feel infantilized by having lists of things they must do:

timetables on sheets of paper as they had at school. Therefore, making these structures as normal as possible is crucial. Ordinary diaries are more acceptable than timetables – the mental health worker manifestly uses one, so it would be quite ordinary for the client to do so. Although it may seem a trivial point, a diary which the person can carry around with them is much more likely to be used than one which cannot, so when purchasing a diary make sure it fits in the person's handbag or pocket, or whatever their normal apparel might be. Prompts can also be made more ordinary and acceptable to the individual, for example an alarm clock rather than a member of staff getting the person up – or even a 'teasmaid'. And they do not need to be given by staff. One client we knew would never get to work if another client with whom he worked did not knock on his door every morning. Telephone prompts can also be useful: in one mental health team where we worked the first task of the morning was to sit and telephone those who had difficulty in getting going in the morning – a sort of 'alarm call' on the NHS! The telephone can also be used to remind a client that you are going to call lest it has slipped their mind.

Regular routines can also be important and this can lead to some counter-intuitive courses of action being beneficial. Often it is assumed that a person who has cognitive and attention difficulties can only manage limited activities, and this may be true. But limiting duration is often more useful than limiting frequency. If a person is expected to engage in an activity on an infrequent basis – say once per week – then it takes a great deal longer to establish the routine. It is often preferable for the person to do an activity daily (albeit for a short period of time), because a daily routine is more predictable and easier to establish than a weekly one.

Often it is assumed that the provision of external structures in these ways will improve the person's concentration and attendance and when it does not we abandon the routine, prompts and structure and assume they have failed. This is a mistake. Even if a person is not able to fit in with the routines and prompts we have devised, the very existence of a structure can have the effect of increasing the predictability of the environment. This predictability can decrease anxiety (for most people chaos is seriously anxiety provoking) and it is known that anxiety exacerbates cognitive confusion and attentional deficits and other problems (e.g. Falloon et al., 1984).

The mental health worker must be prepared to accept that a person may not be able to focus on any activity for very long: they are likely to need a break or to wander off. This must be accommodated without anger or chastisement. However sensitively it is done, telling someone off for leaving early exacerbates their difficulties. On the one hand, they receive the message that they have failed (yet again) and few people will persist with something when they have already failed. On the other hand, even implied criticism can be anxiety provoking, and increasing stress and anxiety exacerbates cognitive problems.

Access for someone who experiences cognitive confusion and attentional deficits can be facilitated by reducing the time for which a person is expected to perform an activity, whether this be a social, work or therapeutic endeavour. All-or-nothing approaches are particularly unhelpful: if a person is required to attend for a whole session or not at all then this may exclude them from the activity. Sometimes simply getting there will be a major achievement, even if the person has to leave immediately. It may be possible to help someone increase the time for which they are able to engage through graded practice: gradually increasing the time for which they perform the activity. Alternatively, a careful examination of what prevents them staying can facilitate the development of ways of circumventing the problems. For example, a person may have difficulty in coping with the social demands of the situation and if they can reduce these within the setting at times when they cannot cope (by going somewhere quiet or going out for a walk) then they may not have to leave. Sometimes a simple system of reinforcers may be effective but it is important to ensure that, at whatever level these are set, the person is able to achieve them most of the time.

Although sometimes it may be possible to increase a person's attention span, often it is not. In this case, acceptance on an ongoing basis that the person will at times only be able to tolerate a few minutes of an activity is important. It does not mean that the activity should be terminated. It may be possible to decrease distractions and stressors within the setting: unplug telephones, arrange for the person to sit on the edge of a social activity without being exhorted to join in. Alternatively, the tasks may be adapted to facilitate short attendance (for example devising work tasks in a sheltered workshop that a person can perform for just a few minutes, or as long as their disabilities allow). Other environmental aids to attentional deficits can be as simple as kettles that turn themselves off and alarms on baths that ring when they are full.

The cognitive demands of social interactions can be decreased. This does not mean talking to the person in an infantile manner but, instead, considering the questions we ask and what demands they place on the individual who is answering them. All comments and questions should be framed in a clear and unambiguous manner, and brevity helps anyone to understand what is being said, complex structures and sub-clauses should be avoided. Repetition and regular summaries can also be important.

General questions like 'What would you like to do?', impose enormous demands – the person has to work out the area of life that is being considered, what all the options are and which of these they would prefer. Multiple choice questions that take into account the person's known preferences – 'Would you like to play football, or would you like to go to the swimming pool?' – impose fewer demands, but rely on the mental health worker already knowing the person's preferences.

It is sometimes easier for a person to follow an argument, explanation or question if it is laid out in a series of points: writing it down can help so that the person can mull it over and has a permanent prompt both within the conversation and outside it. There are numerous areas where written notes can assist communication and circumvent cognitive and attentional difficulties: explanations of what medication does, what problems the person may be experiencing (complete with diagrams of cognitive overload and neurotransmitters), lists of problems they are experiencing for the purposes of monitoring mental state, what is happening in a DSS application.

Sometimes using notes can be an aid to decision-making in a process of 'cognitive chaining'. For example, if the person is being assisted to plan their time, then asking 'What would you like to do today?' may be too complex a decision-making task. Instead, the question can be broken down into a series of smaller decisions – 'What are you going to do immediately after breakfast?, and then?, and then?' – which if they are simultaneously written down assist the person in building the structure they lack. A similar process can also be used for bigger decisions such as what social activities they might like, what they would like to do during the day and where they would like to live. All too often, big questions like these are asked in an 'all at once' fashion under the rubric of giving the person choice. Whether the decisions be big or small, a person's preferences and their right to choose are denied if the process of choosing is not tailored to accommodate their specific difficulties. If a person experiences serious attention deficits and cognitive confusion then decision-making processes may need to be very protracted affairs lasting weeks if not months or years. In each case, the process would follow the structure of a problem-solving cycle: generating a list of all the options available, systematically going through the pros and cons of each, outlining the processes involved in realizing the desired outcome and, on the basis of these, making a decision. A written record of each stage of this process may be an essential basis for the next step.

When conversing with a person who is experiencing cognitive confusion it is often necessary to wait for them to reply. With a disorganized internal world it takes time to process a question, formulate a response and say it. It is tempting for the mental health worker to misunderstand this delay as meaning that the person has not heard the question, or needs further encouragement to respond. However, further elaboration or questioning slows the whole process down even more because the person must then process the new material. It is far better just to wait – however uncomfortable it may feel at the time.

Although the content, duration and structure of interactions and environments are all important, the manner in which interactions are conducted is also crucial. It is very easy to imply that someone is stupid or childlike or in some way responsible for our failure to communicate. The critical rule for all mental health workers must be that any communication failure rests with the practitioner not the client: it is our job to ensure effective communication. Usually, professionals do not 'blame' clients overtly but indirectly imply fault. As Perkins and Dilks (1992) argue, if someone fails to understand what we have said then a statement like 'Do you understand? I'll put it more simply', in effect, renders the client responsible for the communication failure, demeans them by saying that the message must be put more simply. An alternative like

'I'm sorry, I said that in a very garbled way, what I am trying to say is ...' puts the responsibility on the worker for the failure. Similarly, statements that in effect 'test' the person (like 'Do you remember what we did last time?') are not helpful and can make the person feel stupid and inadequate. Giving the information as a matter of course by way of a summary is far more useful ('As you know, last time we discussed ... and decided that ...').

In a similar vein, we have discussed writing things down for clients as a useful strategy, but this assumes that the client can read. Whilst not implying that illiteracy is associated with mental health problems, many clients have numerous social disadvantages that may have impeded their education and some will be unable to read. The stigma of illiteracy is yet another disadvantage that an already disadvantaged group have to bear and many people will be understandably sensitive about it. Once again, in finding out whether writing things down is useful for a client, care must be taken to avoid making the person feel stupid. A strategy that can be useful is to write something down (not type it) and say 'I'm afraid I have awfully bad writing – could you just read that through to check I've written it clearly', or simply to ask them whether they think that writing things down might help.

Consideration needs to be given to everything we do. It is very easy for a chance remark or thoughtless phrase to unwittingly demean or devalue a client. Destructive attitudes about mental health problems are so entrenched within our society that none of us are immune from them. Therefore, continual monitoring of our behaviour is essential.

6

Overcoming the barriers and meeting the challenges

The difficulties clients experience can pose problems in relationship formation. However, the situation is not a one-sided affair. It is important to recognize that mental health workers can, often quite unintentionally, behave in a destructive manner and harbour the unhelpful attitudes that actively mitigate against effective relationship formation and helping people achieve what they want in life. Inevitably, all relationships are complex and at risk of imbalance, over-dependence in one party, abuse of power in another ..., but the relationship between mental health worker and client is particularly susceptible to these problems due to the clients' social disabilities, the breadth of their problems (and the subsequent involvement of the worker in many aspects of their life), their previous experience of mental health services, the duration of the relationship and the fluctuating (but not necessarily improving) nature of their problems and needs.

The goal of effective relationships is to facilitate clients in using their own resources, abilities and strengths to meet their own aspirations and goals rather than the worker making decisions on their behalf, prescribing courses of action, imposing their views or passing judgement. But, as Barker (1992, p. 67) suggests 'We should not lose sight of the fact ... that the more useful we are, the more useless the person might become.'

It is easy for us all to slip into harmful habits or develop deleterious attitudes that impede effective relationships. It is unlikely that anyone who has worked with socially disabled people can say they have never experienced negative feelings towards their clients or behaved in ways that are destructive. In reading the examples that we give it will be easy to think 'I never do that', but such a view is problematic in itself. If we are unable to be critical of ourselves then we cannot be helpful to those who may need our support.

OVERZEALOUSNESS

Overzealous practice refers to workers who are overhelpful: making decisions for the person, taking control of their life, doing for them rather than supporting them to do for themselves. The reasons for overzealousness vary. First, it may arise through understandably being reluctant to give up any part of clients with whom we have developed close relationships. In a genuine desire to be most helpful we may take great pains to develop a meaningful relationship with a person who has previously found it difficult to trust staff. Partly because of this relationship, the person may begin to use other resources and use our support less. However, we have invested a lot in the person and believe that we know them better than anyone else, we are reluctant to allow others to become involved because we fear they might not know the best way of helping this person. Consequently, we discourage the person from broadening their contacts within the service thus meeting our own emotional needs through maintaining the person's dependence, and inevitably preventing them from making choices, developing skills and growing in other directions.

Similarly, we may allow ourselves to be drawn into relationships with clients who flatter us and assure us we are the only person they can really talk to, the only one who can help. Although it may be rewarding to see ourselves as someone's saviour, such a situation is almost invariably destructive for the client. The relationship between client and mental health worker is an unequal, abnormal and circumscribed one. It can never substitute for the rich tapestry of relationships that everyone needs. If the client/worker relationship is to be useful it must actively facilitate the development of other roles and relationships rather than substitute for them. We can never be everything to any individual and nor should we try.

Paradoxically, when we do not make sufficient time for clients, the effect may be similar. Finding out what a person wants from life – what they think and feel, how they see their problems, how and where they would like to live – takes time. The difficulties experienced by someone with mental health problems may make this process more difficult. It can take a long while to make decisions about even such seemingly small issues as what to wear, and even longer to put these decisions into practice. When time is limited and the worker cannot sustain the levels of patience and consideration that might be required there is a great temptation to make decisions for the person: tell them what to wear, identify their wishes and priorities for them, or physically do things for them. It may even appear that doing things for the person improves the result – but in whose terms? Dressing a person may render them 'less scruffy' but it deskills them and further diminishes their confidence and self-worth. It removes the person's choices, undermines any sense of control they may have over their life and may be frustrating and depressing. It is also the case that many of us have very different life experiences from the people with whom we work which inevitably results in different standards, tastes and expectations.

DISTANCING

Regular contact with people who are seriously distressed and disabled and who live in difficult social circumstances, often resenting their need for services and sometimes behaving in unpredictable and unusual ways, places great emotional demands on mental health workers. It is difficult to be constantly aware of a person's needs – and of one's own reactions – particularly in settings that mitigate against the development of support structures and time to reflect and share experiences. Distancing ourselves from people with whom we work is only one of the many forms of defensive practice that result as a means of protecting the member of staff from his or her own emotions. For example, if a person behaves in ways that the we find disgusting or unacceptable it is very difficult to see them as 'like us'. So we emphasize the difference between ourselves and them.

For example, it can be very embarrassing to take someone out who maybe smells or talks loudly about totally inappropriate subjects like defecation or menstruation on the bus. Everyone stares, we feel embarrassed, thinking how dreadful if they assume I am their wife, brother, father or friend. We try in various ways to distance ourselves from them – to show 'I am the nurse and she/he is the patient. They're nothing to do with me, this is just my job.' Perhaps we might instruct them in a loud voice not to talk about those things, treat them like a child in our care for everyone around to see. It is not only in public places that such feelings apply. Even in the privacy of someone's home we may have difficulty in relating to them as an adult, with adult sensitivities and feelings just like our own.

Why are we embarrassed? What does it matter if the person we are with is behaving in ways that we would not choose to adopt ourselves? Why does the way we see ourselves depend on the way someone else is behaving? What must it feel like for the person themself – being stared at, laughed at, avoided? One of us worked with a junior nurse who came back from a drop-in club with a client and said 'They thought I was another patient – kept asking which hospital I'd been in'. 'Congratulations!' was a response that surprised him, but he must have been behaving in ways that reduced the distance/difference between himself and the person he was helping, and this was a good thing.

CLIENT FAILURE

Every mental health worker is pleased when one of the people they are trying to help does well, makes progress. Most of us have experienced the feeling that we too have done well when this happens. We use the achievements of the people we are supporting as an index of our own worth. However, this is somewhat unreasonable: any progress was achieved by the person themself. And there is a reverse side to this coin. As we have seen, people with ongoing mental health problems typically have problems that get worse for periods, as well as better. If the mental health worker's sense of worth and pride in their work hinges on the continued improvement of the people they support, then it is very common to be disappointed and angry when the person deteriorates – they have let us down. The sense of anger and frustration towards the person is very destructive.

Although overt anger is rare we do tend to get fed up, try a little less hard and we may even find ways of blaming the client for their increased problems ('It's not my fault that they got worse, it's because they stopped taking their medication/took drugs/stopped going to the day centre ... They didn't follow my expert advice'.)

Such feelings must be challenged. Do I have the right to claim credit for someone's achievements? Do I have the right to burden them with responsibility for the way I feel about myself? How must they feel about getting worse again? Should I really be feeling angry and wanting to withdraw just when they need me most? Others – family, friends – often reject a person when they are distressed and disturbed, but as the mental health worker our role is to help them through just such times. We might also remind ourselves that fluctuations are in the nature of ongoing mental health problems and try to understand our role differently – as being there during through the bad times as well as the good. If we expect our clients to understand and come to terms with the fluctuations in their difficulties, we need to understand and come to terms with them ourselves.

I'M THE EXPERT

There is nothing wrong with expertise: knowing things, having skills, is a good thing. It is the way in which expertise is used, and the places we look to confirm our expertise, which may be problematic. Most people need someone to tell them that they have skills: expertise has to be acknowledged and confirmed. In the writing of this book we have continually sought reassurance from each other (and others around us) that what we have said is good, right or useful. In mental health work, problems arise if we see ourselves as the source of all expertise and expect our clients to confirm this expertise.

First, it is very reassuring when clients ask us what to do and how do it. It makes us feel we have something to offer. But again, there is a downside. If we always have to be the expert with our clients then we deny their own skills and expertise. If anyone tells us what to do in all situations then we are deskilled. People with serious mental health problems often feel useless – the world has told them they are useless – if we confirm this by being the source of all knowledge then we add to their feelings of inadequacy. Such a situation is destructive because it leads to relationships that further decrease the clients' self-confidence and self-esteem and confirms that they need expert guidance in all matters. However good it feels to be asked for advice we should take a step backwards now and then and ask ourselves 'What are the consequences of giving that advice?', ' Is there another way we could act to help the person to work out what to do themselves?' Would it cost our pride so greatly to say 'I'm not sure – what do you think?' We might fall from our pedestal, but is that such a bad thing if it enables the person to feel their own opinions might just be of value?

Second, there are not inconsiderable numbers of clients who are sick and tired of always being told what to do, and may not take our expert advice. If we expect our clients to confirm our status as experts then when they refuse to do what we say we feel affronted. Sometimes this causes anger – how dare they? Sometimes we decide that they are not worth it – if they won't take our advice/pills/programmes then there is no point in them being here, we may as well discharge them. They are a waste of our resources – better to put our energy and efforts into someone who will 'make use of what we have to offer'.

Challenging these affronted angry feelings in ourselves when someone does not do as we recommend, or indeed does the complete opposite, is particularly important. Not only is such an attitude destructive of relationship formation, it also results in a large number of seriously disabled people failing to get the support and help they need. Why is it so important to us that we 'know best'? Do we always do what 'experts' tell us we should (eat properly, not drink, not smoke ...)? Do we really 'know best'? Have we lived with serious mental health problems? Could we not feel good about letting clients choose what they want to do and supporting them in doing it, even if this is not what we recommend?

THANK YOU

Allied to the problems of expertise are those that arise when we expect our clients to thank us. Britain has a long (and not very honourable) history of drawing a distinction between the 'deserving' and 'non-deserving' poor: those who touch their forelock in an appropriately grateful manner and those who do not. Unfortunately, a similar attitude is not uncommon within mental health services. As mental health workers we like our clients to be grateful for what we have done for them: 'Thank you nurse, you've saved my life' is so much more rewarding than 'Piss off nurse, you've done nothing for me'. If someone is not appreciative of our efforts then it is all too easy for us to resent them ('After all I've done this is all the thanks I get – they don't deserve it.'). It is very easy to withdraw from those who are not grateful for our ministrations in favour of those who are suitably appreciative.

The expectation of gratitude is destructive of relationship formation: like those who refuse to take our advice, those who are not grateful for our ministrations tend to end up being rejected by the services they need (Bachrach, 1989). Challenging such expectations is important. Do I have a right to expect thanks from my clients? With all that they have to live with, can they really take into account my finer feelings? Why are they doing it?

It is worth remembering that the experience of serious mental health problems can be a devastating one and people do not want to need the services they require. It is not, therefore, unreasonable to resent mental health workers as representatives of something they do not want. The hate and anger they sometimes express is typically not directed at us as individuals, but at the system and situation we represent. Maybe the relationship they have with mental health workers is the only one in which it is safe enough to allow the expression of such feelings! A brief glance at the history of many clients shows appalling deprivation and broken relationships. Why should they trust their relationships with us any more than previous ones? Everyone has let them down, thrown them out, rejected them – why should we be any different?

BURN OUT

One of the most frequently cited problems of working with those people who experience serious ongoing mental health problems is that of 'burn out' (Audit Commission, 1994). The work is stressful in many ways: there is always a great deal to be done, risks such as violence and self-harm/suicide are ever present, and individual workers are presented with complicated decisions and situations on a regular basis. However, one of the problems most often quoted is lack of 'throughput': clients failing to 'get better', remaining 'the same'. We have already discussed the way in which all mental health professionals have been trained in cure-based models, expecting to treat clients who get better. These expectations are not met by those with ongoing mental health problems. People can change, and grow, and lead productive and meaningful lives, but they often remain disabled (Birley, 1991).

The reluctance of mental health professionals to work with those with ongoing disabilities has often led to recommendations that services should be 'mixed' so that the staff get to see some movement. Such a model can be disadvantageous to those who have ongoing problems: several studies have shown that, in such situations, staff focus most of their time on more able clients with short term needs (Sayce et al., 1991; Brooker, 1990; Wooff and Goldberg, 1988).

The expectation of 'cure' is destructive of relationship formation because it means that the worker feels demoralized when they cannot see any progress. 'What's the point?' must be something that everyone working with severely socially disabled people has felt at some time. If a mental health worker believes that someone is not 'worth the effort', then enthusiasm and commitment rapidly evaporate.

Challenging such attitudes in oneself can be difficult, because it essentially means finding worth in someone who by broader societal standards is often seen as worthless: they do not contribute to the community via the usual yardsticks of work, family, social relationships. When such a person dies, or kills themself, most mental health professionals will have heard (or been a party to) those hushed conversations amongst their colleagues saying 'It was probably the best thing – they had so little/nothing to live for'. It was such attitudes that led, amongst other things, to the Nazi euthanasia programmes of the 1930s.

Everyone working with people who experience ongoing mental health problems has to find some reason to value those with whom they work or effective relationships and support are impossible and burn out ensues. Such work challenges everyone to examine questions like 'What makes a person valuable?' Different people find answers in a variety of religious and political frameworks, or simple curiosity and a desire to understand the lives of others. Clients often ask 'What is the point?', professionals face a similar question.

FRIENDSHIP

Effective working relationships with people who have serious mental health problems are quite unlike any relationships either within mental health services or outside. They are unlike relationships within acute mental health settings both because of their breadth and duration. The mental health worker has the privilege of knowing about most aspects of the client's life over a length of time that is limited only by their job tenure. This means that the client almost invariably gets to know more about the clinician's life (their moods, the things that happen to them) and there is a temptation on the part of both client and worker for boundaries to become blurred. The client, often extremely socially isolated, sometimes seeks in the worker, who knows the intimate details of their life, the friendship they lack. Mental health workers must be continually aware that clients may be construing their relationship as something which it can never be: friendship, love.

On the other hand, the clinician, after working closely with a client over long periods of time, is not immune from the pull and flattery of such friendship: to be the only person who knows another human being so intimately is tempting indeed. It is therefore quite understandable that workers sometimes transgress the boundaries of a professional relationship. We have known workers give birthday presents, invite clients round for a meal and tell them of their personal difficulties. The difficulties of maintaining 'professional boundaries' can be aggravated by entirely appropriate exhortations to treat clients as the adults they are – with respect and dignity – rather than infantilizing or talking down to them (which is an excellent way of maintaining professional distance).

Mental health worker/client relationships can never be like relationships outside mental health services. Despite the fact that the worker may know more about their client than they do about many of their friends, these relationships can never be friendships because of the context in which they occur. They are by definition unbalanced relationships. The worker is there because they are paid to be there and the relationship exists only because it is the worker's job. The client may be there formally against their will under a section of the Mental Health Act, or informally from lack of anywhere else to be: the worker is therefore both 'jailer' and helper. The relationship is not for the mutual benefit of both worker and client – it is for the benefit of the client and the worker's needs must be met elsewhere.

The worker is in a position of power *vis-à-vis* the client, and however much it may appear harmless, any moves away from working relationship towards friendship constitute an abuse of this power. These abuses are ultimately damaging to the client. The client is burdened with responsibility for the worker's well-being. Favouritism and jealousies too often ensue when one person is given, for example, birthday presents when another is not. Most importantly, the client is let down when the friendship does not extend beyond the duration of the job ('Will you still come and see me after you've left?') or outside of work hours. Friendship may be inviting, but it cannot occur in the mental health worker/client context.

MEETING THE CHALLENGES

The demands of working with people who experience serious ongoing mental health problems can lead to stress in the workers involved. If the negative consequences of such stress are not to lead to poor practice, and destructive relationships with clients, individual supervision and support, and a supportive team and organizational culture, are extremely important.

Clinical supervision

Recent UK DOH recommendations reflect the growing emphasis placed on the support and supervision of all individual workers – a concept most commonly referred to as 'clinical supervision' – which is necessary, whether worker qualified or not. *Vision for the Future* (DOH 1993c) identified supervision as essential to providing effective support, and defined it as:

> A formal process of professional support and learning which enables individual practitioners to develop knowledge and competence, assume responsibility for their own practice and enhance consumer protection and the safety of care in complex situations. It is central to the process of learning and to the expansion of the scope of practice and should be seen as a means of encouraging self assessment and analytical and reflective skills.
>
> *DOH NHSME, 1993*

Supervision refers to a formal process of support for workers to facilitate continued learning and ensure that people using services receive care and support of a high standard. The importance of supervision should be recognized within the team so that time is set aside for each worker on a regular basis. However, its clinical value is likely to be jeopardized if it is linked to managerial objectives like those relating to pay, promotion or disciplinary procedures (Kings Fund Centre, 1995). People are unlikely to reflect usefully upon their mistakes as well as their successes if they feel their supervisor is using this information to assess their competence.

Support, reflection on practice and enhancement of learning may take place on an individual basis or within a group setting. Although the latter option is more economical of time, it does rely on trust and safety within the group so that open and honest disclosure is possible. It is advisable to have an outside facilitator to ensure that ground rules are established, the support function of the group is maintained and learning opportunities are maximized. If supervision is to be conducted on an individual basis the selection of an appropriate supervisor is a crucial consideration. Allowing staff members to select their own supervisors can be successful. Supervisors may come from within or outside the team, they may be from the same discipline or from another, but it is essential that they have training and are sensitive to the particular needs of working with people who have serious ongoing mental health problems.

Each supervisor and supervisee must define the objectives of supervision sessions, and agree on a format. For some people a simple discussion of issues may be appropriate, for others video/audio tapes or written accounts of interactions might form the basis of a reflective analysis, others may prefer to use supervision to plan or rehearse future interactions. The rigid application of a set framework is not appropriate: there has to be scope for flexibility. However, Boud *et al.* (1985) suggest three key strategies that are useful in creating a supportive supervisory environment: exploration, conceptualizing and planning.

1. **Exploration** involves the supervisee recounting particular experiences at length including their associated feelings and thoughts. Supervisor and supervisee identify the skills being used and the ideas, knowledge and beliefs that may have influenced them.

2. **Conceptualizing** may naturally follow on from the process of exploration but has a different intention. The practitioner is encouraged to step back from the experience and develop new ideas and consider alternative constructions of the situation. The aim is to make new connections between the behaviour of the worker and that of the client and to attach alternative meanings to what was happening.

3. **Planning** is a way of supporting the supervisee in working out how to readjust their future client contacts both in terms of beliefs and knowledge and to consider the skills they would wish to use or build upon in further interactions.

This process can encourage skill development and help the worker to anticipate difficulties. It should also recognize limitations and problems that cannot be resolved and consider ways in which these might be accommodated.

Organizational structure

Much has been written about the types of health care settings which mitigate against effective relationships and generate stress within workers. For example, in her classic study in 1960, Isobel Menzies suggested that the organization of nursing services (for example, task-orientated practice and frequent moves between wards and services) was effective in decreasing nurses' anxiety precisely because it prevented ongoing relationships and interactions between nurses and patients. More recently, despite the emphasis placed on consumer choice and quality assurance (DOH, 1989a), increasing managerialism and the drive for cost effectiveness has often limited the time available for workers to have open and flexible relationships with their clients and with one another.

Roles of members of the multi-disciplinary team and their relationships with one another are discussed in detail in the following section. Of most relevance in engendering effective relationships with clients is the culture that exists within the team. An open, sharing and accepting culture, in which workers' relationships with their clients are considered fundamental to the goals of the service, offers a positive basis for good practice. Within such a context, all formal and informal meetings must reflect the centrality of these relationships. Time must be made available to discuss process and progress, share ideas, consider difficulties and seek solutions. This does not mean that consensus is necessary: the skills of mental health work need to be used within the team as well as with clients so that criticism is framed constructively, options for change considered in detail and achievements valued. The environment must be valuing, critical and flexible if bad practice is not to become institutionalized and services developed to really meet the needs of the people who use them.

Overview: Working together

Relationships between mental health workers and clients can only be effective if the worker values and has a genuinely positive regard for those whom they serve, as well as an acceptance of the long term nature of their work. Such relationships must be built on giving people information and support in an acceptable, accessible manner so that they can make and enact their choices and live the lives they want to lead.

On the part of both client and worker, there are numerous factors that can jeopardize relationship formation. Distressing symptoms and experiences can pose problems, as can lack of understanding and dysfunctional attitudes and expectations on the part of the worker. If the negative effects of both of these are to be mitigated then workers must retain an awareness of, and challenge, their own attitudes and beliefs. They must endeavour to comprehend what the world looks like from the position of their clients and explore ways of minimizing the disabling effects of their problems. If it is to be effective, support and help must be based on the individual client's own unique experiences, expectations and coping strategies that they have developed for themselves in the course of living with their serious mental health problems. It is only through carefully listening to people's own stories that mental health workers can gain greater insights into the experience of serious mental health problems and develop new strategies for helping others with similar difficulties.

Effective relationships between clients and workers may not directly change the individuals' situations, but they are central to the delivery of any effective help and support. A valued and trusting relationship is crucial in rendering support acceptable to the person and providing a secure base from which they can explore the possibilities open to them, gain access to the roles and relationships they desire and achieve their ambitions.

The relationship between long term client and mental health worker is an unusual and complicated one because of the circumstances in which it occurs. Without adequate support, mental health workers can look to their relationships with clients for a sense of their own value and skill: take credit for their successes and blame them for their failures with extremely negative consequences for the client. It is not uncommon for the fine line between 'mental health worker' and 'friend' to become blurred. The roles of client and worker and the power imbalance inherent in the context in which the relationship occurs renders this inappropriate and dangerous. Attractive as the notion of friendship might be, it is not an option in this context.

In place of friendship, mental health workers can be **allies** to their clients. Often people with serious mental health problems are relatively alone in a hostile world. Unlike so many other people in their lives, mental health workers can provide an ongoing relationship that can be trusted through good and bad times alike. We can be on the side of our clients: helping them to do the things they want to do, to carve out a life for themselves, develop friendships and relationships and take risks, knowing that we will make ourselves scarce if they do not need us but always be there when things go wrong. In short, instead of abusing our power in relation to our clients, or denying that we have it (as has become fashionable), we can use it as their allies.

PART THREE

Contexts of Support

Introduction

People who are seriously disabled by ongoing mental health problems require support in a variety of areas of their lives. In former times this would have been provided by nurses and direct-care staff in institutions with intermittent input from psychiatrists. Moves away from this institutional system have been accompanied by changing philosophies of care and increasingly complex systems and contexts of care.

There is an increasing range of workers involved in providing support. Psychologists, social workers, occupational therapists, community care assistants, drama and art therapists, welfare rights workers and support aides, some of whom have a history of mental health problems themselves, have joined nurses and psychiatrists in providing assistance. In addition, probation officers, teachers, families, local housing officers, employers, community workers, friends and neighbours might be involved. Although this multi-disciplinary and multi-agency network offers a breadth of expertise and range of skills, it is not without problems in day to day practice. The roles of the different people involved and the way in which they work together to provide support for individuals are of great importance.

Support is provided in an increasing range of settings: apart from outreach work taking place in the person's own home and community, direct care may be provided in specialist hostels, group homes, staffed houses, supported flats, sheltered workplaces, drop-in facilities, day centres and community mental health centres. Development of the internal health care market and specific recommendations to purchase non-statutory care services (DOH, 1989a, 1990a) have increased the range of agencies providing this support. Thus, a variety of social services, voluntary sector, private and jointly funded residential, work, social, leisure and therapy services have been added to the traditional Health Service provision. These different agencies and facilities have different priorities and methods of day to day running as well as different funding arrangements, but effective coordination between them is vital if individuals are to receive the support they need.

Inevitably, people's needs and wishes change, services open and close, and people with long term mental health problems have to move from one setting to another. Such moves can be distressing and problematic for the individuals concerned. It is therefore important to minimize the disruptive effects of change in the context in which the person receives the assistance they require.

Multi-disciplinary and multi-agency working

7

The deleterious effects of practices occurring in psychiatric institutions have been widely documented (Barton, 1959; Goffman, 1961; King *et al.*, 1971). Although the practices that developed in institutions were designed to facilitate the smooth running of those institutions, many are perpetuated in community-based facilities through the good – but misguided – intentions of staff working there. Evidently, changing the location of support does not automatically lead to a more client-orientated approach (Brown *et al.*, 1966; King *et al.,* 1971; Ryan, 1979; Allen *et al.*, 1985). If they are to benefit clients, moves away from institutional care must be accompanied by a similar departure from the damaging institutional practices that were characteristic of such places. Goffman (1961) described the key features of such institutions.

1. **Institutions are total in that residents work, sleep and spend their leisure time in the same place.** The totality of institutions is perpetuated by a desire to ensure that people get all the services they need. Inevitably, this is most easily and rigorously ensured if all day and leisure activities are available in a person's place of residence. Yet, whenever this occurs, that place of residence tends to become a total institution. Difficult and time-consuming as it may be, it is important to provide people with the help and support that they need to engage in different activities in different places. Playing bingo in the local bingo hall, for example, rather than in a group bingo session in their hostel/hospital, or going to the General Practitioner's surgery rather than have a doctor visit them.

2. **Institutions are segregated from everyday social life and residents have little contact with the world outside.** One consequence of totality is the creation of segregated communities of people who are disabled by mental health problems and whose members have little contact with those who are not so disabled other than the staff who are paid to provide their care. The

stigma of mental health problems can make 'the community' an uncomfortable place for those who do not always look and behave in the expected manner. Segregation is often justified on the basis of minimizing the abuse and rejection that people with mental health problems too often experience. Yet, if such segregation is perpetuated then non-disabled people remain ignorant of the needs and problems of their counterparts with mental health problems, and those who are disabled are denied access to the ordinary social contacts, activities and opportunities that are their rights as citizens. Stigma and discrimination can only be diminished if we make efforts to render our communities accessible to, and accepting of, people with serious mental health problems.

3. **Institutions have rigid routines and an overall plan guides even the smallest details of people's lives.** Although such routines undoubtedly assist the smooth running of an institution, they are often initiated as an efficient means of ensuring that everyone gets the help that they need. Whilst most people have routines, they are routines that the individual tailors to their own needs and wishes, and they can be broken when necessary. For example, whilst we may usually do the washing-up before we go to bed at night, we may break this routine and leave it to the morning if we are tired after a hard day or if our friends stay late. Meals in hospitals and hostels too often happen at set and immutable times, day in day out, and washing-up must be done immediately afterwards. It is not always easy to allow flexibility of routines, especially in communal living situations, but it is essential if the negative effects of institutionalization are to be avoided.

4. **Institutions are regimented and employ block treatment.** The same rules and practices tend to apply to everyone irrespective of their needs. Where people live in a group that is not of their choosing, as in a hospital, hostel or group home, efforts to individualize care and support are often thwarted because of notions of fairness ... and block treatment results. Arguments such as 'It is not fair for John to lie in bed all morning if Mary has to get up at 8 am to go to work' and 'It is not fair for James to have his washing-up done for him if Mark has to do his for himself' effectively prevent the tailoring of support to the individual's needs. Ironically, the one area in which such 'fairness' arguments are rarely proffered is that of medication. If someone said 'It's not fair that she gets stelazine when I only get chlorpromazine' it is unlikely that the mental health worker would have any hesitation in responding that different people have different problems and therefore their medication is different. The same arguments must apply to all areas of help and support if it is really to be tailored to each person's needs.

5. **Institutions are depersonalizing.** Patients are not treated as individuals and they are deprived of the rights and status of ordinary people. In our society there are few models of how to behave towards those who experience the

thinking and feeling difficulties associated with serious mental health problems. People with such problems are often treated as children in need of care and protection: helpless beings who must be protected and on whose behalf decisions must be made. Whilst such protectiveness may result from the best of intentions, when a person is overprotected, deemed incapable of making decisions for themselves, their personhood is removed: they are deskilled and devalued.

6. **In institutions there is a large social distance between staff and residents.** This may be manifested in many ways, including uniforms and separate, staff-only, toilets, mugs and cutlery. Often staff find it difficult to share spaces and materials with clients who may not have the standards of hygiene and behaviour that they demand, but what does this say about the way in which they view those whom they are supposed to be helping? The degradation implied by deeming clients unfit to share a toilet or use the same cutlery and crockery as staff is enormous. Furthermore, the perpetuation of such distinctions calls into question the standards of care provided by the staff: if a cup or a toilet is not sanitary enough for staff to use, can it be said to be adequately clean for clients?

In general, if the destructive social distance of institutionalization is to be avoided then there must be a transformation in the way in which help and support are provided. Supervising and observing people and doing things to them must be replaced by being with them and doing things with them. As everyone knows, being in need of help and support to do things that most people appear to manage unaided can be a belittling and devaluing experience. This is made worse if there is a large gulf between the helper and the helped. People with serious mental health problems are no different from anyone else in this regard, except that through years of having been deemed helpless and incompetent they have often, quite understandably, lost confidence in their abilities. For anyone, it is easier to give assistance than to receive it and we feel stupid if we are always on the receiving end of help from others. Support is both more palatable and more valuing of the person if it is provided by someone working alongside them deciding what to do and doing it together. To be directed by a distant expert who tells them when they do things wrong or does things for them is a confidence-sapping experience.

7. **In institutions, residents have little control or say over what happens.** All decisions are made by staff. Often it is assumed that because people have cognitive and emotional problems they do not know what is best for them. Staff are the experts who are employed to know what is good for the client and they are failing in 'their duty of care' if they do not tell clients what to do. The notion of choice is valued highly in the western world, a value that is shared by those who have been deprived of such choices because of their mental heath problems. To be deprived of choice and control over what happens to us is a destructive and devaluing experience.

Although the choices available to every citizen are constrained, the deprivation of choice and control that occurs in mental health services often goes well beyond the considerations of resources, legality or safety imposed on all citizens. For example, one of us recently attended a meeting where the residents of a residential unit were being given a choice of the colour that the walls should be painted ... but they were only offered a choice of delicate pastel shades. The staff were fearful that residents would choose something inappropriate: perhaps they would want the ceiling painted black or choose colours that clashed. The concept of choice is only meaningful if a person, whether they have mental health problems or not, has the right to make 'wrong' or 'bad' choices. It is difficult to stand by and watch someone make bad choices and there are times when it is disastrous to do so. But preventing colours clashing is hardly equivalent to preventing a person from jumping under a bus.

8. **Residents in institutions are deprived of normal social roles and have little opportunity to engage in ordinary, everyday activities.** The roles of mother, father, lover, worker, are replaced by the devalued 'patient role'. The patient role may be appropriate and useful for relieving a person of responsibilities during brief periods of sickness: it may be appropriate to take to one's bed and be looked after for a while when one has influenza. But when the patient role becomes a way of life – as it so often does when a person has ongoing disabilities – it is extremely destructive, restrictive and degrading.

It is often very difficult to help someone take up a variety of social roles when they are generally considered to be incapable of meeting the demands of such roles by virtue of their mental health problems. When someone has been deprived of ordinary roles and activities for a protracted period it is not surprising that they lose confidence in their ability. Anyone who has been out of work, or who has not driven a car for a prolonged period, knows the crises of confidence, apprehension and anxiety that resuming the role of worker or driver entails. They also know the importance of having others around who understand their fears and have the confidence in their ability to succeed that they themselves lack. It frequently falls to mental health workers to believe in the person's abilities and to provide the supportive and encouraging relationship that is necessary if ordinary role functioning is to be resumed.

People with serious ongoing mental health problems have multiple needs that span both social and health domains. It is therefore inevitable that they will require assistance in a variety of areas from a range of sources. The provision of comprehensive support has to be seen as a collaborative affair bringing together the expertise and experience of different individuals, agencies and the client him/herself. Such joint working is not easy because of the different values and priorities of different people and agencies, the difficulties involved in consistent and continuous communication, and the fluctuating nature of the individuals' needs and wishes. It is not surprising that confusions, gaps, and conflicts arise and cause problems for the individual and workers involved.

THE MULTI-DISCIPLINARY CLINICAL TEAM

Collaboration is essential for the provision of effective mental health services which can meet the broad and disparate needs of people with serious mental health problems. Most mental health teams comprise a variety of professions – typically, nurses, psychiatrists, psychologists and occupational therapists who work alongside social workers employed by the local authority. The advantages of such a multi-disciplinary mix have been identified by Muir (1984) as:

> ... the opportunity to pool skills and share work by using the specialist knowledge of team members, gaining wider professional awareness of problems of the client group, exploring a variety of potential solutions to problems, understanding the role of other professionals, and the giving and receiving of support.

Their disadvantages include:

> ... having to work closely with people you may dislike or not agree with, spending time in lengthy meetings where efforts may be directed towards group maintenance rather than towards the task, individual initiatives being hindered by pressures towards group conformity, and less contact with clients because of team demands.

The roles of the different professionals who make up the mental health care team vary and any description is likely to be hotly debated. However, stereotypical accounts of the philosophical and practical differences between different professionals often suggest greater barriers than those actually found in practice (Fishe, 1984). Each professional brings to the clinical setting a variety of skills. Some of these are the core skills of their profession, others are additional skills they may have acquired through formal training or experience and it is not uncommon for there to be an overlap in skills between professions. For example, whilst cognitive and behaviour therapy are core skills of a psychologist many nurses may have gained specific training in these techniques.

In addition, there are a whole range of personal attributes, not directly related to the mental health setting, that individual workers may bring. Gender, age, race, sexuality, class and cultural backgrounds, and the different experiences that these entail, can all be important in the process of relationship formation and the provision of long term support. In ensuring that different individuals who have serious mental health problems can gain access to the communities that are relevant to them, an understanding of these diverse communities is vital. It is not only the client, but the team as a whole, who can benefit from the range of cultural backgrounds of its members. Finally, workers may have other skills, unrelated to their mental health expertise. For example, a mental health worker who is also a musician can use these skills to perform meaningful and valued musical activities with clients. Interests can also be important: for example, if a client is interested in football, or racing, interaction with a worker who shares their interests can enhance the person's self-worth and the process of relationship formation.

In the context of the different cultural backgrounds and skills that each individual brings to the mental health setting, the core areas of expertise for each professional might be summarized as follows.

Psychiatrists have an expertise in the assessment of mental state and symptomatology, and the control of this through psychotropic medication. Many will have an understanding of the relationship between social factors and psychiatric symptomatology as well as training in other psychological and family interventions.

Clinical psychologists have an expertise in psychological models, assessments and interventions. They engage in a variety of cognitive, behavioural and psychodynamic interventions with individuals, groups and families. They may provide expertise to other professionals concerning ways of maximizing a person's strengths and the effects of different interventions based on psychological theories and research. Psychologists have specific training in research and data collection, therefore they will often be involved in monitoring, evaluation and in developing systems of team working.

Occupational therapists typically provide a range of social, leisure and, sometimes, work activities. They have an expertise in assessing where a person's performance has broken down and in skills training and development, as well as support, to enable the person to make the best use of their abilities. In relation to physical disabilities that people who have mental health problems might also experience, occupational therapists have expertise in determining the aids and environmental adaptations that a person may require to make the most of their skills.

Social workers are generally concerned with the individual's interaction with the world outside psychiatry. This may include finding places where a person might live, work, or spend their leisure time, work with families to enable a disabled person to regain or maintain their role as part of the family unit, and work with the disabled individual to enable them to take on a variety of social and family roles. Social workers may also take a role in helping people to obtain the benefits to which they are entitled and may be trained in a variety of specific therapies.

Nurses still provide the majority of direct care within mental health services, although they are being joined by a range of mental health support workers, housekeepers and residential social workers. Nurses, as well as these other groups, have the major role to play in the actual delivery of treatment and care – whether this be the provision of medication or help with day to day life, the organizing of activities, providing counselling, advice and a listening ear, or simply being there to share a person's distress. Increasingly, nurses are gaining specialist skills in a range of therapeutic interventions.

Whilst these are the most frequently occurring professions within psychiatric teams serving those who have serious ongoing mental health problems, it is important not to forget that there are a variety of other professionals and services within the psychiatric enterprise who provide vital expertise and services.

Arts therapists. Some people with mental health problems have difficulty in articulating their feelings, difficulties and dilemmas. Art, dance and movement therapists can play a role by affording a therapeutic medium that does not rely on verbal abilities.

Analytic psychotherapists. Many people who experience serious ongoing mental health problems cannot take advantage of analytic psychotherapy itself – frequently they lack the 'ego strength' necessary for the success of such interventions. Nevertheless, analytic models and understandings of an individual can be useful, especially when other professionals are feeling stuck or at a loss about how to understand why the person is behaving and reacting in the way that they do. Such models can enable the team to view a person in a new light.

Pharmacists. Most people with serious long term mental health problems are taking psychotropic medication, and many have received a vast array of different pharmacological and physical interventions. Pharmacists have an in-depth understanding of the range of medication available, the research literature concerning these, the side-effects and the consequences of different dosages and combinations of drugs. This can be important in advising mental health workers and their clients, and in ensuring that people receive the optimum medication for their problems.

Welfare rights advisers. Poverty is extremely common amongst people who experience serious ongoing mental health problems: a person's disabilities are greatly aggravated by having to live on a pitifully small income. The under-claiming of state benefits is frequently reported by welfare rights pressure groups and can be particularly common amongst people with mental health problems. Negotiating the benefit system is a complex task that requires much patience, tenacity and understanding. The long telephone calls, waiting and persistence required often prevent those who have serious cognitive and emotional problems gaining access to that which is rightfully theirs. Most mental health workers are not welfare rights experts and therefore are not in a position to properly assist their clients. The benefit systems requires that the expertise of dedicated welfare rights experts can ensure that people get all of the benefits to which they are entitled. Further, the advice of welfare rights experts can be vital in establishing residential facilities and work programmes that do not financially disadvantage those whom they are designed to serve.

Legal advice. Many people with mental health problems require legal advice from time to time – either in relation to detention under the Mental Health Act or with other more general problems. Community legal facilities do not always have the expertise necessary to help: advice and representation in relation to the Mental Health Act is a specialist field and representing someone who has cognitive and emotional problems requires an understanding of the social difficulties that these can cause. Access to specialist legal advice can be achieved either by setting up independent, specialist Legal Advice projects within mental health services or by providing training and advice to existing community facilities.

Patients councils and advocacy groups. People with mental health problems sometimes find negotiating the complexities of psychiatric services themselves a difficult and daunting task. It is not uncommon for new and more junior staff to have difficulty in expressing their opinions within the organization. Therefore, it is hardly surprising when clients have problems articulating their wishes and feelings about the service they are receiving. Many clients have had bad experiences in the psychiatric system and as a consequence do not trust the professionals involved to act in their best interests: they are likely to have experienced many situations in which their views have not been heard or taken seriously.

For these reasons, people need access to independent advocacy: someone who they trust to be on their side and help them to get their views across. Sometimes this takes the form of 'citizen advocacy' – someone from outside the psychiatric system who has not had mental health problems to be with the person and speaking for them. This has the disadvantage of perpetuating the belief that people with mental health problems cannot speak for themselves. In enhancing the esteem and respect of the disabled individual, and ensuring that they are assisted by someone who really understands their situation, a preferable model is that provided by Patients Councils and User Advocacy Networks. These can offer both individual and group advocacy that is trusted by services' users because it is provided by others who are, or have been, in the same position.

There is much that the range of individuals, professions and services within the psychiatric world can do to support people who are seriously disabled by ongoing mental health problems. However, the aim of working with such people is to enable them to gain and maintain access to their communities and the roles, relationships, activities and facilities therein. Therefore, in considering multi-disciplinary and multi-agency working, it is essential to look outside the hospital, mental health service or Community Mental Health Team.

BEYOND MENTAL HEALTH SERVICES

Recent years have seen explicit policies to encourage a 'mixed economy of care' and a diversification of care providers (DOH, 1989a, 1990a). Broadly these can be divided into those whose explicit remit is to provide support and shelter for people with mental health problems, and those ordinary individuals and agencies who provide services to the whole community.

Services specifically for people who have mental health problems are provided by social services, voluntary (not for profit) organizations, the private sector and volunteer agencies. Social services provide a multiplicity of day, residential, social and, sometimes, employment facilities. Flexibility and variety can be increased if they also fund services jointly with either voluntary sector, or health, services (Howat et al., 1988).

The voluntary sector has had a role in providing accommodation for people with mental health problems that stretches back to the end of the last century and the Mental After Care Association (Wing and Morris, 1981). Today there are numerous local and national voluntary agencies providing various kinds of hostel and supported accommodation. The growth of special needs housing provided by Housing Associations means that much of the accommodation for people with serious mental health problems is provided within the voluntary sector. Voluntary sector provision also includes day, work, drop-in and social facilities.

The major role for the private sector has been in the provision of residential care and nursing homes (see Perkins et al., 1989a, b). Such accommodation has often been widely (but not exclusively) used in providing alternatives to hospitalization for elderly old long-stay patients: those whose continuing needs relate more to the frailty of advancing years than to the mental health difficulties that resulted in their hospitalization decades before.

Volunteers have been involved in mental health services and facilities in a variety of capacities. Most hospitals have volunteers helping out with a number of social and leisure activities, but probably their major role has been in befriending. People with serious ongoing mental health problems are often extremely socially isolated and befrienders may be used to make up for the friends they do not have. Sometimes these befriending relationships can be extremely effective, but they can create problems. Although many befrienders are reliable, the unpaid nature of the role can lead to it not being taken seriously: befrienders may not come when they say they will come or may drop out of contact. Some see their role as 'saving' the person from psychiatric services – undoing the damage they believe such services to have wrought. This is inevitably in conflict with others who provide support and the disabled individual is pulled in opposite directions. Yet other befrienders may be intent doing their bit to help 'poor unfortunates' – hardly the basis of a good validating relationship with the 'poor unfortunate' concerned. It is therefore important that befrienders are carefully selected and trained, and alternative models do exist. In Montpelier, Vermont, there exists a different model of befriending which involves service users themselves acting as buddies for people with similar problems who are socially isolated. This model provides much needed social contacts as well as providing appropriate role models and makes active use of the buddies' experience of mental health problems to assist others with similar difficulties (Perkins, 1993).

NON-SPECIALIST HELP IN THE COMMUNITY

There are various people and agencies who have a role in the support of people with mental health problems whose remit is not specifically geared to provide for this group. The families of socially disabled people often have an important role. Families provide a great deal of the basic personal and social care of their disabled members (Perring et al., 1990) and often fail to receive the support that they need in so doing (Norbeck et al., 1991). A disabled individual's family and friends are important whether or not they are living together. They can form a large part of the disabled person's social networks: a vital link with the community and the world outside the mental health arena that is easily lost over years of service use, through neglect and lack of support. Fostering and rebuilding these connections can be critical in ensuring that a disabled person's access to their culture and community is maintained.

General Practitioners often have a role to play in the delivery of maintenance medication and support, but physical health care must not be overlooked. Often people who are seriously disabled by long term mental health problems have physical health difficulties that are not diagnosed/treated (Koran et al., 1989; Wells et al., 1989), and it is not uncommon for them to fail to receive routine physical health care screening (Perkins and Fisher, 1995b).

Local authority housing departments often have contact with those who experience mental health problems. On the one hand, they have to find suitable temporary and permanent housing for such people when they have nowhere to live. On the other hand, they have to respond to the concerns and complaints of other tenants when a disabled person is behaving in ways that disturbs others. In addition, local authority home care services can provide vital help with domestic chores, shopping, meals, paying bills, collecting their benefits from the Post Office and alerting others when things are not going well, help that is so necessary in enabling many to live in their own homes.

Religion and spirituality are as important to many people with mental health problems as they are to others in the community. Churches, synagogues, temples and various religious leaders provide not only religious and spiritual support but also social contact and a community to which the disabled person can belong.

The police have a high level of contact with those few people with serious mental health problems whose behaviour is disruptive or disturbing to others in the community. Police involvement is most widely documented in relation to compulsory detention and transport to a 'place of safety' under Section 136 of the 1983 Mental Health Act (Rogers and Faulkener, 1987), but there are other ways in which they have a role in supporting people with mental health problems. For example, such people can be vulnerable to assault, attack and robbery (Bachrach, 1985), and neighbourhood policemen/women are often in a position to keep an eye on them to ensure that they are not harmed and to alert services if they suspect problems. In another role, some people who experience cognitive and emotional problems contact the police repeatedly, either because they believe they have committed offences or that others have offended against them. The police require support and education so that they can respond appropriately and better help this section of the community whom they serve.

The list of agencies, people and facilities in local communities who have a role in supporting those with mental health problems is almost endless: it varies from area to area and person to person. It may include neighbours, shopkeepers, landlords, sports facilities, community centres, citizens advice bureaux, cinemas, chemists, Post Offices, bingo halls and launderette attendants. To give some examples from our own clinical experience. One man always had his lunch in a particular café – this provided him with important social contacts as well as food. If he did not appear it almost invariably meant that something was wrong. Therefore, the café owner would alert the mental health team if he failed to show up. A woman had a similar arrangement with the proprietor of a local pub where she could invariably rely on one of the customers buying her a Guinness each lunchtime. Another woman liked to spend time in the Post Office watching people come in and out and chatting to them as they did so – the Post Office manager provided her with a chair because, at the age of 70, she found standing for too long very tiring. A young man was extremely interested in philosophy and mysticism and did not like any of the available mental health day facilities. He had little to do in the day until he found a local health food shop with whose proprietors he could discuss his theories, and where he was allowed to help out for a few hours each day serving and advising on various alternative remedies.

The contact that these people had with community agencies was vital in many ways: providing social contact, structuring their day, enabling them to engage in ordinary, meaningful activities and providing an early warning when difficulties arose.

In any community there will be numerous agencies and activities for people with different interests and backgrounds. The aim is to enable a disabled person to gain access to those that are relevant to them. It is therefore vital that workers know about, and maximize the use of, all opportunities available. Whilst it may be easiest to identify those facilities and activities specifically for people with mental health problems, use of these means that the person remains in the segregated world of mental health problems: they may be in the community but they are not part of it. Segregated facilities do have a role: they can provide specialist help and afford people the opportunity of being with others who have experienced the similar difficulties. However, if a person **only** uses segregated resources they have less opportunity to develop other facets of themselves: to be something other than a person with mental health problems. In effect, two communities are created – one for the able-minded and one for the socially disabled – neither of which can benefit from the skills, talents and understandings of the other.

Where specialist facilities and activities are needed it is possible to decrease their segregation by ensuring that they can be used by both people with mental health problems **and** those who do not have such difficulties. Sheltered employment in the form of shops serving the general public offer one such opportunity, as do cafés and drop-in centres. Even old hospitals can offer much needed space for activities and meetings of local groups, thus ensuring that people from the local area share spaces and places with those who have mental health problems.

In 1968, Criswell defined rehabilitation as helping the psychiatrically handicapped person and the non-handicapped person to live together. If this is to become a reality then two things are important. First, people with social disabilities must be enabled to use ordinary facilities and engage in ordinary roles and relationships within communities. Second, people without social disabilities must be helped to understand and accommodate those who are disabled. In order to achieve both of these aims close liaison between the mental health workers and other agencies is vital.

In helping a disabled person to use ordinary facilities and engage in ordinary relationships it is necessary for the mental health worker to know what is available in the local community that might be of interest to the clients concerned and to understand the demands and constraints of these situations. They must support the individual in line with these demands and constraints so that they can use their strengths and minimize the disruptive effect of their disabilities. This support may be transitional, but equally it may not: it must be provided for as long as it is needed and available whenever difficulties arise.

To assist people without social disabilities to accommodate those who have such problems, it is necessary for the mental health worker to help them to understand the nature of cognitive and emotional problems and, in particular, to understand that whilst the person may have some problems they are not universally disabled, or stupid, or lazy, or bad: an ability to appreciate the person's strengths, assets and abilities is vital. The person/agency must be provided with the support they need in order to accommodate the disabled individual. This could be anything from someone to accompany the person in the activity (whether this be going to visit parents, going to an aerobics class, visiting a night club, or going on a Gay Pride march), to education in how help might best be provided and someone to call if difficulties arise. Ongoing liaison, advice and practical help with difficulties are important to maintain access: they must be provided for as long as they are required.

This support is necessary whether the 'agency' in question is the person's family, their friends, their general practitioner, a religious group, the housing department, the local day centre or anywhere else. Community contacts rarely 'just happen', they need to be actively promoted, fostered and supported.

8 | Collaboration and coordination

There are many potential advantages of multi-disciplinary, multi-agency work but problems can arise. Such difficulties include practical considerations relating to the coordination of care and deciding upon who does what: role blurring and role differentiation within the multi-disciplinary team and across agencies. They also include differing philosophies and models, and the jealousies and destructive competitiveness that can arise.

When people who were seriously disabled by ongoing mental health problems lived, worked and spent their leisure time in the hospital it was relatively easy to ensure that what support they received was coordinated, but the degradation, segregation and institutionalization inherent in such settings were a high price to pay. The shift to community-based care has been accompanied by a proliferation in the agencies and people involved in the support of each individual and coordination of care has become a big issue. Two major problems can arise: gaps in the provision of care and duplication in care.

Gaps in care generally mean that the person fails to receive the support they need because everyone thinks that someone else is doing it. Such omissions can occur in any area, for example, monitoring a person's mental state and picking up signs of relapse: the community nurse thinks the hostel staff are doing it, the hostel staff think the GP is doing it and the GP thinks the community nurse is doing it.

Duplication of care is not only costly in terms of scarce resources, it can also be costly in terms of confusion on the part of the client. For example, the psychiatrist and the housing support staff may both be talking to the individual about their medication. The psychiatrist may be trying to help the individual to understand that medication is keeping them well and that they will probably have to take it for a very long time, whilst the housing support staff may be saying how well the person is doing and that if they carry on the way they are they will probably be able to reduce and eventually stop taking the drugs altogether. There are numerous occasions where, because different professionals or agencies have different models or perspectives, they are giving the individual contradictory advice.

CARE PLANNING

In order to avoid both gaps, duplication of support and contradictory messages, clear, coordinated care planning is essential. Such care planning is a major cornerstone of current UK mental health policy (DOH, 1990a, b, 1991) and requires several elements. First, a thorough assessment of the individual's wants, wishes, needs and problems is required. This involves all those who have contact with the person. No one has a monopoly of knowledge: different people see different facets of the individual, therefore the views of all concerned must be incorporated, including and especially the disabled individual him/herself.

All parties must negotiate and reach an agreement concerning the major directions – long term goals – towards which support will be directed. If we do not know the direction in which we are heading it is not possible to design appropriate care/support in the short term. The agreed care plan is directed at helping the person move towards these longer term goals. It should outline all the input that the person will receive and who will provide it. A named individual (keyworker, care manager, named nurse) must be identified, this person is responsible for ensuring that the care plan is coordinated and enacted in practice.

Over recent years care management has been hailed as the answer to all the problems in providing services for people disabled by mental health problems. Although care management has many advantages, it is not without shortcomings. At its least, care management offers the individual a named worker to assess their needs and to implement and monitor their care, coordinating the input of all appropriate agencies in line with plans made at regular review meetings (Repper and Peacham, 1991). This provides a central point of contact for all those services involved in supporting the individual and, more importantly, for the individual him/herself it ensures that one person holds overall responsibility for their support (Repper and Cooney, 1994).

Essential to the success of care management is the relationship between care manager and the person receiving support. It is only in a trusting relationship that the client is able to contribute meaningfully to their own care plan and express their feelings about the services they are receiving (Repper et al., 1994). Thus, proper care management refers to more than a mere configuration of services, but to an approach towards working with people who experience serious mental health problems. In this form it has been demonstrated to be more effective than traditional means of service organization in engaging clients in services and in maintaining contact with them – reducing drop-out (Ford et al., 1995).

However, the effectiveness of care management depends upon a range of public services, residential, day and outreach care being available (Shepherd,

1990). However skilled he/she might be, a care manager alone cannot be expected to provide all the ongoing support, care, education and treatment that a person may require. Given the multiplicity of a disabled person's needs, it is unlikely that any one individual or agency could possess all the necessary expertise. It is therefore important for people with a range of skills to contribute to a comprehensive system of supports and implement appropriate care.

If people who are seriously disabled by ongoing mental health problems are to receive support that optimizes their strengths and allows them to do the things they want to do, then a partnership is required between the individual concerned, people who understand the various facets of their emotional, cognitive and behavioural difficulties, and people who are expert in providing help and support in each area of need. To give an example: we worked with a man who was in his early 20s. In addition to his serious cognitive and emotional problems, he had a history of becoming violent to others when the 'voices in his head' became too bad. He was a very able man who wanted to study for a GCSE in English. Helping him to achieve this involved a collaboration between his psychiatrist, named nurse, psychologist and a tutor at the college. The tutor provided information about what would be required for him to take an English course – how many sessions he would have to attend, what he would have to do in these sessions and what would be required between sessions. With this information, the psychiatrist, psychologist and the nurse collaborated to assess, through direct observation and specific assessments, where he would be likely to experience problems. This involved not only consideration of such areas as his concentration and attention span, but also of his violent and disruptive behaviour: the situations that were likely to trigger these, the warning signs and ways of preventing problems occurring. This analysis enabled the psychologist and nurse to help the man to practise and prepare for the classes, and to liaise with the college tutor about areas in which he might experience difficulty and things she might do to help him. The nurse arranged to help him to get to the classes – initially going with him, but then simply providing prompts and reminders as his confidence grew. The nurse also remained in regular contact with the tutor to resolve difficulties as they arose. He passed his English literature GCSE and is now trying to decide whether next to embark on Art or Geography.

The young man had defined what he wanted to do. Different members of the multi-disciplinary clinical team offered expertise concerning the ways in which his problems might impede his wish to begin studying again and how these difficulties might be circumvented. The tutor from the local college provided expertise in the teaching of English literature and the demands upon students. Bringing these areas of expertise together enabled him to achieve his ambitions.

There is a tendency within care management for a person with serious ongoing problems to actually see only one member of the multidisciplinary team – the care manager – who receives advice from other experts. This can be problematic. First, it conveys to the disabled individual the inaccurate message that a single person can be the font of all knowledge: they never see the help that the care manager gets from others. It can be unhelpful for someone whose self-confidence is already at a low ebb to be presented with an individual who appears to be omnicompetent. It is more realistic for a client to see that those who provide their support have limitations themselves and do not always know the answer. Second, although a single worker may be able to gain some expertise in areas with which they were not familiar, they are unlikely to be able to gain an equivalent competence to that possessed by someone who specializes in that area. This means that they are unlikely to be as creative in their application of that knowledge or as adept at problem solving when things do not go as planned. For example, a support worker may receive some background training on welfare benefits, but they are unlikely to have the breadth of understanding that a welfare rights expert would possess.

Third, many seriously disabled clients are extremely socially isolated. If they have contact with only one worker then they have the opportunity of only one relationship – and this in itself is extremely limiting. Most of us have the opportunity of being different things to different people: to be responsible, competent and assertive at work, to be pathetic and incompetent with our nearest and dearest, and to be radical, delinquent and sometimes irresponsible with our friends. Most people have access to a wide variety of roles. Each of these roles allows them to manifest different facets of their character and interests, and each of them supports the others. If we had not the opportunity to express our fears and insecurities at home, and to gain the support and reassurance of our loved ones, it is unlikely that we could be competent and assertive at work.

It is very difficult for both client and worker to adopt different roles in relation to each other in different situations. Different situations demand different behaviours. If the same worker is involved then inappropriate behaviour can be encouraged on the part of both worker and client. If a worker who, in hospital, helps the person with their personal hygiene also goes to the pub with them, there is a temptation for the worker's hospital role to extend to the social situation. He/she may, for example, tell the person to tuck in their shirt, or blow his nose, both of which might be inappropriate in a pub. The situation can be equally difficult for the client. If he/she is used to talking about problems, personal issues and medication with a worker in their hostel, then it can be difficult for them to refrain from this usual behaviour when they are in a social or leisure role outside: talking about incontinence is simply inappropriate on a bus! Role confusion on the part of both worker and client can be decreased if different workers engage with the client in different roles and situations.

If people with serious ongoing mental health problems are to make the best use of their abilities and skills, and realize their ambitions, then it is helpful for them to have the opportunity to be different people in different situations. A person may talk about their problems, symptoms, uncertainties, insecurities with their nurse or doctor, but they also need the opportunity to be a valued and competent worker, friend, son, daughter, spouse, lover, in settings where their symptoms take second place. Different roles and relationships have different demands and allow the person to be something other than a 'psychiatric patient': contact with different professionals, agencies and individuals is vital, both within and outside the psychiatric milieu.

ROLE BLURRING AND ROLE DIFFERENTIATION

In a multi-disciplinary, multi-agency setting there can often be conflict about whose job it is to provide different aspects of support. As we have already outlined, there are some areas which are the special expertise of people with particular professional training. To the extent that the professional training of mental health workers differs, role differentiation occurs. So, for example, it is the psychiatrist's job to prescribe medication, the psychologist's to carry out cognitive therapy and the nurse's to give an injection. On the other hand, probably the majority of the support that a disabled individual requires is not clearly within the professional province of anyone. Whose job is it to provide supportive counselling, help the person to get to the bank, clean out their fridge or help them shop for food? To the best of our knowledge, fridge cleaning and shopping do not form part of the training of any mental health professional, but they can be highly skilled exercises. We have already considered the skills involved in helping someone without making them feel stupid or deskilling them: offering them assistance in an acceptable, non-degrading manner. In any continuing support setting there will be a great deal of role blurring. There are many, very necessary, forms of support that do not fall within the specific remit of a particular profession and could be carried out by many different people.

Within teams and between agencies numerous disputes can arise concerning role differentiation and the specific skills associated with specific professions. Similar disputes arise concerning who should do those things that do not fall within the specific professional competence of any one agency or individual. It often seems to be the case that those interventions that have a high status (treatment, psychotherapy, counselling) are claimed as the specific responsibility of many professionals (Patmore and Weaver, 1991). For example, psychiatrists, psychologists, counsellors, nurses, social workers, housing support staff, day centre staff, occupational therapists, may all claim an expertise in counselling and psychotherapy. On the other hand, those activities that have historically had a lower status (helping someone to get up in the morning, cleaning, shopping, getting to the Post Office) are often deemed to be 'not my job' by everyone concerned.

Such demarcation disputes are destructive of effective support, especially as those basic activities of everyday life that carry a low status are also those that are often most central to a person's community survival. In order to avoid destructive demarcation disputes two factors are important. First, it is necessary for everyone in the team to have a clear understanding and respect for the roles of different professionals and agencies, and second, a culture that explicitly elevates the basics of everyday life from their lowly status in the professional world and accepts both their central importance and the skilled art involved in their delivery. In such an environment all professionals and agencies should be willing to place the clients' needs at centre stage and engage in some of those tasks that are considered 'less desirable', in addition to work within their narrow professional area. All aspects of the person's care should be thoroughly addressed in multi-disciplinary, multi-agency reviews so that there is a shared understanding of the range of needs of the individual and a general commitment to ensure that these needs are met.

JEALOUSIES AND COMPETITIVENESS

Different workers and agencies have a history of antipathy towards each other, as Kingdon (1992) suggests 'differences in status and renumeration between groups have been usually unspoken factors impeding collaboration'. Typically, each believes that they know what is best for 'their' clients and often base their judgement of other professions or agencies on inaccurate generalizations. So, for example, psychiatric teams may believe that the voluntary sector consists of a group of libertarians with unrealistic notions about mental health problems whilst voluntary organizations may believe that psychiatric services damage people with drugs and institutionalization. Psychiatrists may reject the socio-political stance of social workers whilst social workers may hate the drugs and 'medical model' of psychiatry. Whilst many of these are caricatured attitudes, there are numerous vestiges of such views that colour relationships between professionals, agencies and local communities.

Probably one of the most problematic areas is that of the closure of old psychiatric hospitals and the transfer of former residents to other facilities in the community. Nurses and other care staff in the old hospitals often feel personally criticized for the care they have offered over the years and see their jobs disappearing as the hospital runs down. Those in the community facilities can often be heard to talk of the 'institutional attitudes' of staff in the old hospitals and it has often been stated that the old hospital staff should not transfer to new community facilities because they would bring their outdated attitudes with them.

Such competitions and jealousies are extremely destructive of inter-disciplinary and inter-agency cooperation and detract from effective care and support for those clients whom they serve. Often the disabled person finds themself the object of a bizarre kind of 'tug of love' with numerous different people purporting to know what is best for them.

Overcoming what is often a long history of antipathy can be difficult. Where multi-disciplinary mental health teams have been working together for some time, many of the old rivalries have been broken down. However, there often continues to be a mutual suspicion between different agencies. If such rivalries are to be avoided it is essential that all the individuals, agencies and professionals involved get to know and value each other's work, perspectives and views. Mutual understanding can often go a long way to breaking down suspicions and misunderstandings.

DIFFERING PHILOSOPHIES AND MODELS

Philosophical differences can cause great problems in multi-disciplinary working. Sometimes these differences are more implicit than explicit and their effect is even more marked because they cannot be discussed and debated. Classically, there has been a divide between what has been called the 'medical model' and just about everything else. Adherents of the 'medical model' are supposed to believe that mental health problems are an illness, that all of a person's problems result from this illness and that the only 'cure' (if cure is possible) is to be found via drugs and other forms of physical treatment. In opposition to this there are a plethora of psychological and social models that variously argue, for example, that what is called mental illness is an understandable reaction to adverse social and material circumstances, or a consequence of distorted communication patterns within families.

Often disputes revolve around whether the 'medical model' is 'true' or not, and this is extremely unhelpful. The 'medical model' – or, more properly, an extreme organic perspective – is something of a straw man to which few psychiatrists would adhere. It has long been recognized and demonstrated by psychiatrists themselves that, even if one assumes some organic pathology, this does not mean that social factors are unimportant, or that all of a person's problems can be accounted for in terms of the organic pathology. Different models are likely to be important in understanding different facets of a person's behaviour and experience, and it is very likely to be the case that an understanding of physical, neurochemical, psychological and social factors is important in understanding the range of human experience in any sphere.

Although different values, beliefs and ways of working can result in bitter disputes between workers and contradictory support across agencies and providers, they do not have to be destructive. The presence of differing philosophies and models can increase the options available, generating new ways of viewing a person's difficulties and alternative means of providing them with support and help. It is neither possible nor desirable for everyone to adopt the same perspective on mental health problems. However, if differences are to be constructive, rather than destructive, then it is important that philosophies and models are made explicit so that they can be openly discussed and understood. All members of the team must accept that it is possible to understand anything in a number of different ways. Different models may be appropriate for understanding different problems. It is entirely possible to believe that some of a person's problems result from neurochemical abnormalities, whilst others result from a disrupted childhood and/or other social and material disadvantages. It is also possible to adopt one model for understanding problems and another for alleviating them: it is still possible to adopt social interventions to alleviate cognitive and emotional difficulties even if it is believed that the cause of these lies in the neurochemical domain.

The choice between these different theories and perspectives should be made in terms of their acceptability to the client concerned and their utility in helping them to achieve what they want to achieve. It must be accepted that clients have models and theories too, and that they are most likely to accept those types of intervention that make sense within their own models of what is happening to them (Perkins and Moodley, 1993a, b).

Socially disabled people have little to gain from rifts and irresolvable differences between the agencies and individuals who provide them with support. The 'guild disputes' between different professions and agencies that have long characterized mental health services may seem very important to the professionals involved, but they are largely irrelevant and destructive to clients. A person who requires help does not care whether the psychiatrist, the psychologist or the nurse leads the mental health team but they do need support to be provided in a respectful and dignified manner in order to achieve what they wish to achieve.

Moving from one place to another

The proliferation in locations and agencies providing support for people with serious ongoing mental health problems sometimes brings with it a necessity for these people to move from one place to another to get the support that they need. On the one hand, changing patterns of provision mean that people who have historically been provided with support solely in a hospital setting have to move to other locations. On the other hand, the support needs of an individual change over time: this may necessitate moves between different locations and providers. Over a one-year period in the long term care service in which one of us works, 30% of people living in community settings required at least one admission to hospital or a period of intensive day support.

Moving from one place or service to another can be a difficult and disruptive process, but there are many ways in which the need to move can be reduced. In general, the principle should be that, unless there are clear reasons to the contrary, it is preferable for support to move to the individual rather than for the individual to move to the support.

RESETTLEMENT

Resettlement refers to a person moving from one place to another – quite literally, settling again. It might best be conceptualized as one amongst many possible ways of helping a person to pursue their ambitions and interests, gain access to social roles and relationships, and minimize their handicaps. Frequently, resettlement is taken to mean the process of moving where someone sleeps at night from a hospital to a non-hospital facility. However, it also involves moves between different living, working, social and leisure environments, and moves between different hospital or community facilities. Examples of resettlement would therefore include: moving from a hospital Industrial Therapy Unit to a community sheltered workshop; from a community sheltered workshop to open employment; from a parental home to a hostel; from a hostel to an independent flat; from one hospital ward to another; from a community setting to hospital; from the hospital physiotherapy weights room to the local gym; from the day centre social evening to the local community centre; from playing bingo on the ward to the local bingo hall or from shopping at the hospital shop to the local stores.

Resettlement of any kind involves a series of major life events: moving house, changing job, leaving family and friends, changing leisure and spare time activities, and coping with a new set of roles and expectations. There is now an extensive literature showing that major life events are distressing and have a deleterious effect on the health, well-being and functioning of anyone (Nezu and Ronan, 1985). A moment's reflection will provide ample anecdotal evidence of the trauma and miseries involved in moving house, changing job, getting married, getting unmarried, changing partners, losing friends. For someone who has serious ongoing mental health problems, these effects are magnified. People with such difficulties often have problems in coping with day to day life unaided and can be particularly vulnerable to the effects of life events and changes that other people take in their stride. The stressful effects of changes can manifest themselves in a deterioration in ability to cope with everyday situations, behavioural disturbance, exacerbation of cognitive and emotional problems, and acute personal distress. There is now a well-established body of evidence that shows a link between life events and the onset of depressive episodes (Brown and Harris, 1978), schizophrenia (see Falloon and Fadden, 1993) and mania (see Ambelas, 1979, 1987).

It is important to acknowledge that apparently minor changes can have a devastating effect upon someone who is particularly vulnerable by virtue of their mental health problems. Anyone who has worked in a continuing care setting will have seen distress and deterioration of functioning in the face of such things as staff changes and changes in routine. Even rumours of change can be deleterious. Recently we have seen a worsening in the behaviour, day to day coping skills and symptoms of three people following a rumour that everyone was going to move to a community-based house.

Moves and changes can cause three types of problems. First, they can result in increasing difficulty coping with day to day life and worsening cognitive and emotional problems. Often it is possible to provide increased support and help over the difficult period of move until these transitional problems are alleviated. However, the deterioration may be so severe that the person cannot be accommodated in the setting to which they are to move. For example, a woman with whom we work functions extremely well in a hospital setting. She looks after herself, can cook and clean, and has a clerical job in one of the hospital departments – she is certainly competent enough to cope outside hospital and often goes to the local social services asking for somewhere to live. However, she is extremely vulnerable to the deleterious effects of even the slightest hint of change. Despite a high level of support, on each occasion that a move has been suggested her behaviour and mental state have deteriorated dramatically. She has damaged a great deal of property (throwing chairs through windows etc.), become extremely violent towards other residents and staff, ceased to wash and care for herself, taken to her bed, and engaged in much self-injurious behaviour. This extreme reaction effectively makes her 'unplaceable'. Although it is probably a transitional response, there exist no facilities in the district that can cope with her violence and self-harm, and provide the intensive staff input needed, even for a short period of time. She has the skills and competencies to cope outside hospital but in practical terms it has not been possible to enable her to effect the transition.

Even if a person's temporary deterioration over the transitional period is less severe, a second problem arises because it is often impossible to predict when transitional problems will occur (Perkins *et al.*, 1992). One man was so disturbed by the initial suggestion of a move that he required continuous observation for over a week, but then gradually improved, moved without difficulties and has been happy ever since. Another younger man was happy with the initial idea of moving, but as the time approached he became increasingly distressed and it was only intensive support that enabled him to move. One woman welcomed the idea of moving but immediately upon taking residence outside hospital became doubly incontinent for several weeks. Another became distressed and anxious from the time she heard about the move until around one month afterwards, when she settled and was fine.

Finally, the deleterious effects of change and major life events are extremely aversive for the individuals concerned. In trying to avoid personal distress someone may therefore be extremely reluctant to undergo changes that cause them misery and anxiety. This can raise enormous practical difficulties for resettlement and pose ethical questions about the concept and reality of choice.

CHOICE AND RESETTLEMENT

If a person says they do not want to move should we accept this at face value? How many of us have wanted to change our job, but when the moment comes – when we have to say goodbye to all our old colleagues and clients – have wanted to change our minds and to stay if it were possible? Similarly, when moving house – leaving one part of the country and moving to another – we would almost certainly have said no if anyone had asked us if we wanted to move at the point of actually moving. The reality is often that people find the **process** of change aversive – want it all to be over or wish they had never embarked upon it – but do want the **outcome** of the changes (more money, a better job, a bigger house). Unfortunately, it is impossible to separate process and outcome. In asking someone whether they want to move, particularly someone who is vulnerable to the deleterious effects of change, the answer conflates process and outcome. If the process is too daunting then a person is likely to say they do not want the change even if they do want the outcome of that change.

This confusion can cause people to appear inconsistent in their choices. Sometimes they say they want to move, sometimes they say that they do not. It is too easy to assume that this ambivalence reflects the intrinsic unreliability of someone with mental health problems and to interpret it as meaning that someone else must make their decision for them. But this is inaccurate. Every human being, whether disabled or not, simultaneously holds differing and often contradictory views. For example, people may hold religious beliefs and simultaneously believe in scientific explanations which are incompatible with their religion. Choice is important, but when contradictory preferences are expressed we must help a person to come to a resolution.

Giving someone a choice about moving is often seen as a simple task: telling them the options and asking what they want, or asking questions like 'Where would you like to live?' or 'What job would you like to do?' without giving any information about the range of options available. If anyone is asked big questions like these in such a decontextualized way, then they are likely to opt either for that which they know (their existing home or their existing job), or some extension of this (a higher grade in the same job, a bigger house in an area they know), or to give a fantastic answer that they would probably not want to be committed to when it came to it (to become the Prime Minister or live in a French chateau). Yet we do make choices about our lives and the question is how we can ensure that people with mental health problems have similar choices. In order to do this we need to think about choice in a more sophisticated way.

For most people, real choices are severely limited and often it is the **belief** that there is a choice which is important rather than the reality of whether these choices can actually be exercised. Choices are limited not only by personal and material constraints, but also by other choices a person has made. The making of one choice rules out other possibilities. For example, if someone decides on one career others are obviated. If someone has a partner, then the location in which they live and work is limited. Everyone has limited choices, but people who have serious ongoing mental health problems often have fewer real choices available to them, and fewer personal and social resources with which to make those choices. Choices are usually limited by poverty, prejudice, other social disadvantages and the availability of the support needed. The ability to make choices is also limited by restricted knowledge and experience of the options available, as well as cognitive and emotional problems that render more difficult the process of actually making choices. In addition, many people lack the confidence to make decisions for themselves. Years of having decisions made for you, having your opinions and views disbelieved and dismissed, exacts a high price in terms of your faith in your ability to choose. If the possibility of disabled people making choices over how they live their lives is to be maximized then all the issues associated with giving a person real choice need to be considered carefully: awareness of the real options available, what these options might be like, help to weigh up the pros and cons of difficult possibilities and support to realize the alternatives selected (see Chapter 4).

STRATEGIES FOR MINIMIZING THE DISRUPTIVE EFFECTS OF RESETTLEMENT

It will probably never be possible to completely obviate the disruptive effect of moving in whatever domain it occurs. The longer a person has spent in their existing setting, the more difficult a change is likely to be. Even if someone has actively chosen a particular move, this does not mean that it will be unproblematic: as we have described, the process of change is likely to be difficult even if the outcome is desirable. However, there are several ways in which the disruptive effects of changes can be minimized.

First, it is important to give the person time and support to get used to the idea of moving and come to terms with the losses it involves. Any change inevitably involves giving up some things and taking on new ones, and giving up something, particularly when it is something that you have known for many years, is a bereavement. This bereavement occurs even if the person intensely dislikes their existing setting.

Second, it is sometimes important to prepare the person for their new setting. However, our experience has shown that there are enormous individual differences in this regard that should be heeded. Some people like to jump straight into a swimming pool or rip a sticking plaster off all in one go. Others prefer to let themselves into the water gradually or peel off a plaster bit by bit. Similarly, some people prefer a prolonged period of getting used to the idea before they actually take the plunge whilst others like to think about the move as little as possible.

It is usually sensible to do as much preparation in the new setting as is possible to avoid generalization and transfer of skill problems (Shepherd, 1977, 1978). For example, it is often possible to take a person to what will be the local shops and Post Office several times before they move in order to familiarize them with their new surroundings. However, care should be taken not to prolong the preparation period unnecessarily as anticipatory anxiety can increase, undoing some of the benefits of the early familiarization. Furthermore, the person can come to believe that the move is simply not going to happen. Other people find preparation for a move extremely anxiety provoking and avoid all preparatory activities, as one young man said to us 'Don't worry, I'll go when the time comes, but I don't want to think about it until then'. He moved out of hospital two months later with no difficulty.

Third, it is important to prepare the placement for the individual. All too often, preparation for a move is seen in terms of changing the individual to fit into their environment – a process that often involves a great deal of training in, for example, shopping, cooking, cleaning and managing money. Although some skills training may be necessary, we have already discussed the shortcomings of an exclusively skills-based approach (see Chapter 2): the main task is ensuring access. In terms of resettlement, this means changing the place to which the individual is going so that it can accommodate them and their needs. This can often involve negotiations with a variety of agencies and individuals to form a network of continuing support **before** the person moves. Further, it is probably sensible to beware of 'honeymoon effects': it can be the case that over the immediate period of a move people's functioning improves but after a few months returns to its original, pre-resettlement level (Perkins *et al.*, 1992). It appears that some people require less support outside an institutional setting, some require more, and others require about the same (Perkins *et al.*, 1992), and there do not appear to be good ways of predicting this for any one individual. It is probably most sensible to assume that, overall, the same level of support will be needed, with a flexibility to cater for individual differences as they arise. In preparing a placement for an individual, it is also important to consider the attitudes and understanding of other people in the community to which the person will move. The deterioration in public attitudes towards people with mental illness (Scottish Association for Mental Health, 1992) is increasingly impeding the development of community facilities for people with serious mental health problems.

Fourth, it is important to anticipate and contain any deterioration in cognitive and emotional problems and ability to cope, and the increased distress that may arise: it is not uncommon for someone to require additional input, support, tolerance and understanding during the process of moving. Sometimes, such a deterioration is seen as an indication that the move would be inappropriate for the individual. This is not always the case. It is entirely possible that it is the process of moving with which the person is having difficulties, rather than the place to which they are moving. To abandon the move because of a temporary deterioration may disadvantage the individual concerned.

Fifth, in any resettlement it is important to maintain as much continuity as possible. A single move can actually involve several major life events and the more changes there are the more difficult and distressing the move. Minimizing the number of changes that a person has to undertake can be achieved if, for example, the person moves house but is able to continue to use familiar day, outreach or social facilities after they have moved. Alternatively, the person can commence new work, day or social activities and get to know new staff before they move.

PUBLIC ATTITUDES: ISSUES AND RESOLUTIONS

The nature of media coverage of mental health issues means that attention is directed towards facilities which are seen to be problematic (Rabkin *et al.*, 1984), whilst those which have developed smoothly and without resistance receive little or no publicity. The absence of problems must be the norm as 99% of people with mental health problems now live in the community (Mental Health Foundation, 1989). Nevertheless, public resistance towards the siting of projects for people with mental health problems in or near their own communities is becoming more common and increasingly powerful (Glass, 1989; Dear and Gleeson, 1991; Dincin, 1993). In the past 10 years, the Mental After Care Association (MACA) have set up 35 houses for people with mental health problems, but it is only in the past three years that they have experienced problems with local residents that have sometimes threatened the siting of projects (Bynon, 1994). The Scottish Association for Mental Health also reports an increasingly negative response in some neighbourhoods. This has threatened the viability of several projects and has led to their withdrawal in one case (Scottish Association for Mental Health, 1992). It is important to note that 'the public' who object to developments for people with mental health problems includes mental health workers: Dincin (1993) described a situation in which psychologists led local opposition to a supported housing development.

The arguments most frequently expressed in opposition to mental health projects reflect three main concerns (Dear and Taylor, 1982; Solomon, 1983; Dear, 1990; Wenocur and Belcher, 1990; Dear, 1992). First, the perceived threat to property values. Although this is a common source of opposition to the development of new projects (Boydell et al., 1989), careful research has consistently found that property values have not been affected by mental health developments (Dear and Taylor, 1982; Boydell et al., 1989).

Second, concerns about personal security. Such fears are often expressed in questions about the supervision of clients. They are more common if clients are perceived to be dangerous or unpredictable, including those people with serious mental health problems (Dear and Gleeson, 1991; Dear, 1992). Third, the perceived threat to neighbourhood amenities. Local businesses and residents worry about the impact of antisocial or unkempt people upon the quality of the area.

The extent of public opposition appears to be influenced largely by four factors (Segal and Aviram, 1978; Sundeen and Fiske, 1982; Dear and Wolch, 1987; Glass, 1989; Dear, 1992). The proximity of the facility: the closer the facility is to their own home, the more vociferous the opposition. The clients who will be using the facility: drug addicts, offenders and people known to have a psychotic diagnosis are perceived as most threatening. The size and visibility of the facility, and the community in which it is situated: closely integrated, middle-class communities are more likely to mount effective opposition than mixed or marginalized communities.

In order to promote effective relationships with the local community the size, function and implications of the proposed facility must be taken into consideration. Since neighbours would not be informed about a large family moving into their street, it contravenes the principles of normalization to inform neighbours about the use of a house for people with mental health problems. However, neighbours can be helpful and constructive when they feel involved (Segal *et al.*, 1980). Therefore, it is not always clear whether it is best to inform and consult them from the outset or to respond only if opposition arises. The practical experience of the Mental Aftercare Association suggests that informing the local population of a proposed project immediately provokes anxiety and concern. They have found the least conflict evoking strategy to be a low profile, no information approach, followed by direct and personal contact – in their own home – with people who complain (Bynon, 1994).

Our own experience suggests that people with serious ongoing mental health problems are their own best advocates. Therefore, much of the preparation involved in this regard entails introducing the individual to their new neighbours, workmates or other people engaged in social or leisure activities. However, it is often the case that some education is necessary to dispel the myths about mental health that so often abound and support for others in the situation, especially someone to call when things go wrong. To give two examples from our own experience.

In one project, several people hospitalized with serious mental health problems wanted to use a local community centre that offered drop-in facilities and numerous activities. The centre was contacted and initially expressed some concerns about the disruptive effect such people might have and about their inability to offer the necessary support. Mental health service staff talked to centre staff about mental health problems and provided literature about the sorts of difficulties that people experienced. After a while the centre staff said how unfair it was that such people should spend all their days stuck in a psychiatric hospital and, of course, they would like them to use the centre ... but only if they were accompanied by staff. This was agreed, but it was not long before the centre staff began to ask why the mental health staff were going with their clients to the centre. It was agreed that mental health services would continue to provide transport for clients and the centre staff were given a number which they could contact in the case of problems. At the time of writing this arrangement has been working well for five years and many disabled people use the centre alongside their non-disabled counterparts. There have been one or two problems (including aggressive behaviour and incontinence) but when contacted mental health team staff have always been quick to respond.

In another project, neighbours initially objected to the establishment of a community house in their street. They variously argued about danger to their children, property prices and the danger posed to disabled residents by proximity to a major London football ground. Several community meetings were held, but the anxiety of residents was not full assuaged and letters to the MP continued. The immediate neighbours were invited to tea with the future residents and the meeting went well. All residents in the street were given a telephone number so that they had the security of knowing that they had somewhere to call should problems arise. Four years on problems have arisen on only two occasions when residents held parties that caused some noise disturbance.

Issues relating to the public attitudes towards people with serious ongoing mental health problems are important in many areas. The extent to which individuals with such difficulties can gain access to the roles, relationships and activities that make up communities will in part be determined by the attitudes that prevail in those communities. In the early days of resettlement it was generally claimed by service providers that people with mental health problems were 'no different' from anyone else. This was probably a well meaning, but naïve, mistake. It led to a situation in which people with mental health problems could be members of communities only insofar as they could 'act normal' – be closeted about their disabilities. Whilst the needs, wants and aspirations of disabled people are no different from those of any other citizens, their rights as citizens must include the right to be members of communities with mental health problems. It would obviously be extremely oppressive to argue that people with physical limitations could only be accommodated in non-disabled communities if they could behave as if they were not disabled. The growing number of regulations governing disabled access are testimony to the campaigns of physically disabled people for adaptations to the non-disabled world to allow them access. Such access requirements rarely encompass those who are socially disabled by cognitive and emotional problems, but the situation is the same: access to communities cannot be restricted to those who can pretend they are not disabled.

Overview: Demarcation or delivery?

Everyone involved with someone who experiences serious mental health problems, from the nurse and the psychiatrist, through to the local authority social services department, the GP, family, friends and neighbours, all have an important role. It is necessary to move away from the position that particular kinds of interventions and help are in some way better, or more important, than others. It is not the case that medication, counselling and psychotherapy are more valuable than helping someone collect their benefits and get food. These latter activities have long been the preserve of direct care workers and families who have often received little acknowledgement of the importance of their efforts.

Irrespective of status, within teams and agencies it is those people who have greatest contact with the individual who will have the greatest role in determining the quality of service that they receive. The simple existence of a coordinated plan does not ensure that a person actually gets the support they need in the manner in which they will accept it (Perkins and Fisher, 1995).

Wherever a person lives or works, whether they need to move or can be helped to stay, whatever their diagnosis or level of disability, the critical issue is how to ensure that they receive the support they need, for as long as they need it, in a manner that is acceptable to them. This will depend upon the quality of relationship with the care provider, upon services being flexible and non-time limited, upon priority being given to their choices and their very individual needs and strengths, and to attention being paid to the preparation of communities to facilitate access. Often it is known what would help the individual to make the best use of their skills, the critical issue is whether this is delivered. Smallpox was not eliminated by the discovery of a vaccine but by ensuring the universal delivery of that vaccine to people. The same is true in relation to mental health problems. We may not have many 'cures' as such, but a great deal is known about interventions and support that can alleviate problems – the critical issue is how we deliver these to the person who needs them. Any care plan or intervention will stand or fall on the skills and actions of those people who actually provide the support and care and their skills in delivering these in ways that are acceptable to the person concerned.

PART FOUR

Specific Therapeutic Interventions: Helping People Cope

Introduction

Until relatively recently, interventions to help people who experience serious ongoing mental health problems were largely restricted to drugs, asylum and practical help with day to day chores. When asked what they find most helpful, people with such problems cite the friendship of those members of staff who actually talk to them, share their experiences and appear to enjoy spending time with them (Johnson, 1995). Despite this, until recently, counselling and psychotherapeutic approaches have not been pursued with those who have serious cognitive and emotional difficulties. There appear to have been several reasons for this.

First, people with serious mental health problems are often said to have 'lost contact with reality' and as such would not understand any kind of talking therapy. They may be difficult to engage in conversation and so it is assumed that they would not be able to respond within a counselling framework. They may be deemed to 'lack insight', which may be taken to mean that there is little point in listening to what they say because the content of their speech is simply a reflection of their psychopathology. Clearly, if it is assumed that what a person says is not worth taking seriously (except as an index of their mental health problems) then talking therapies would not be worth while.

Second, the way in which serious mental illness was understood effectively prevented the development of psychotherapeutic interventions (Bellack, 1986). For many years schizophrenia was conceptualized as a biological disorder which could only be treated by drugs and which by definition would not be amenable to psychotherapy. Similarly, the anti-psychiatry response that schizophrenia did not exist further inhibited the development of psychotherapeutic interventions.

Third, it has often been observed that people with serious mental health problems lack the 'ego strength' supposed to be necessary for the traditional insight-oriented psychotherapies (Bachrach, 1982). Along similar lines, people with such problems have difficulty in coping with the closeness and pressures of intensive psychotherapy, and such approaches can be actively destructive by increasing the person's cognitive problems.

Finally, on a more practical note, those professionals who typically provide 'talking therapies' – psychologists, psychotherapists, counsellors, social workers – have had limited input into services for people with serious ongoing mental health problems. If a person's problems are ongoing then by definition cure-based interventions are relatively futile.

Over the last 30 years, however, this situation has changed. Interest initially focused on behavioural approaches which dealt primarily with overt behaviour rather than internal experiences, beliefs and feelings. Thus, token economy systems and other behavioural approaches were developed to reinforce behaviour that was considered to be adaptive (Allyon and Azrin, 1968; Gripp and Magaro, 1974, Kazdin, 1978), to decrease problem behaviours and develop skills in a variety of areas (Anthony, 1977; Wallace, 1989; Liberman *et al.*, 1986; Jacobs *et al.*, 1992).

Dynamic psychotherapy has rarely been utilized in its pure form with those who have serious mental health problems in mainstream service settings (Berke, 1979; Menn *et al.*, 1975). However, some of the principles of psychotherapy were introduced in the treatment of the families of people with a diagnosis of schizophrenia. Brown *et al.* (1958), Brown (1985) and Vaughn and Leff (1976a, b) identified the deleterious effects of familial critical comments and emotional overinvolvement on the individual. Subsequently, a number of people working in the field have developed therapeutic strategies for working with families to reduce the likelihood of the disabled individual relapsing and to reduce the stress on the family (Leff and Vaughn, 1985; Leff *et al.*,1985; Birchwood *et al.*, 1992; Tarrier, 1992; Falloon and Fadden, 1993).

During the early 1980s, concern focused upon ways in which psychotherapy could be rendered appropriate for people who had traditionally been excluded because of their serious mental health problems (Bachrach, 1982; Stewart, 1985). In particular, such authors argued that in order to be most effective, a problem-solving approach needed to be adopted, based on the 'here and now', or present situation of the person. Thus, people with such problems could be helped to understand the effects of stress on their difficulties, develop ways of dealing with this and so gain control over their lives.

Latterly, interest has expanded to include helping people to develop strategies to deal with their cognitive and emotional problems, monitor and modify their own symptomatology and minimize the likelihood of relapse. The effectiveness of these interventions has been demonstrated in terms of clinical and functional improvements and subjective satisfaction (e.g. Chadwick and Lowe, 1990; Tarrier *et al.*, 1988; Birchwood and Tarrier, 1992).

Medication and behavioural approaches | 10

Since the 1950s, when the effects of phenothiazines on the symptoms of schizo-phrenia were discovered, drug treatments for serious mental health problems have taken precedence over other forms of help. Although many other social or psychological interventions have since been developed, these are almost invari-ably combined with pharmacological treatment. Whilst drugs may have a contribution to make, it has become clear that other approaches are necessary. In the 1960s psychologists began to develop behavioural interventions, most notably the 'token economy' approach (Allyon and Azrin, 1968).

Both pharmacological and behavioural approaches remain controversial, probably because they are seen as 'doing things to' the person – in the form of chemicals or external reinforcement contingencies – rather than enabling them to take control of their own lives. Whilst it is undoubtedly the case that both medical and behavioural regimes have been abused, the extreme positions taken by their proponents and opponents are not useful. Both have a role to play in minimizing a person's disabilities and enabling them to live the life they choose, but neither is the panacea that they have been claimed. Their role, where they have one, must be seen alongside other interventions and environ-mental changes to facilitate access for disabled people.

MEDICATION

There is no medication that can 'cure' any serious mental health problems, but there are an increasing number of drugs available that can alleviate and control some of the symptoms. These drugs do, however, have serious side-effects: in considering the appropriateness of medication for any individual, it is essential to weigh the therapeutic benefits against the costs. Medication must be consid-ered in the context of the aims of supporting someone who has long term mental health problems. Throughout this text we have argued that the main aim should be to enable people to have access to roles, relationships, activities and facilities within communities so that they can make the most of their skills and abilities and achieve their aspirations and ambitions. Where a person's symptoms are extremely distressing and debilitating they often welcome medication as a source of relief. As one woman said '... they stop the strain on my brain'. However, where side-effects make a person feel awful, look odd and render them unable to perform in social roles they can actively impede access.

Probably the biggest issues in relation to medication revolve around power, choice, information and consultation. All too often, professionals prescribe psychotropic drugs with little consultation and discussion with clients about the effects, side-effects and options available to them. Sandford (1994) asked people who attended depot clinics for their views about their medication: most of them felt they had been given poor reasons for having their injections, many felt they received too much medication and substantial numbers reported receiving little information about side-effects. Choice and power rest with the professionals not the clients.

Sometimes professionals have a legal right under mental health legislation to assume such power. However, in the majority of instances, mental health professionals are accorded such power not by law but by the structure and operation of mental health services which renders users relatively powerless. The information and power imbalance between users and providers is such that recipients have to accept that which is offered to them or receive no help at all. Luckstead and Coursey (1995) found that 30% of service users reported having been pressured into taking medication – and the most common type of pressure used was verbal persuasion.

In this context, it is important to distinguish between discussion, the giving of information and persuasion. In most services it is probably true to say that when medication is prescribed for a person the prescribing doctor talks to the client about the drugs they are giving. However, the nature of these discussions rarely takes the form of consideration of the various options open to the person, the effects and side-effects of the medication available, and the advantages and disadvantages of taking it so that the client can make an informed decision about whether they want to take the medication or which medication they would prefer to try. Similarly, there is rarely a consideration of what it will feel like to take the drugs prescribed. This means that the client is placed in an all or nothing position of accepting the doctor's view on the subject and taking the pills or rejecting it and getting nothing (other than the risk of compulsory detention). The power afforded mental health professionals by both their position in services and their access to information means that if they choose to persuade a client to take medication the client will generally agree, and even if the client does not really agree there are other sanctions that professionals can employ to ensure that the person 'takes their advice'.

If a person refuses to take the prescribed medicines then they are frequently deemed 'non-compliant' and ways of 'increasing compliance' are considered.

In addition to 'prompting' and 'encouragement' (which outside a mental health service would too often look like nagging and bullying), it is not uncommon for residence in a particular hostel, attendance at a day or work programme, or receipt of other forms of care, to be made contingent upon the taking of medication: '... if you don't have your injection you cannot live here ...'.

Whilst there are undoubtedly times when someone is not able to make decisions about what happens to them, these times of acute distress and disturbance are almost invariably time limited. If the medication has the desired effects it should render the person able to make decisions about it and decisions about whether they wish to continue to take it. It is also possible to discuss with the client their views and preferences in relation to medication (and other forms of help/treatment) when they are in a less disturbed period. A 'crisis plan', previously agreed between the client and the worker, can give people more control over what happens to them at times when they are unable to make such choices.

People who have serious ongoing mental health problems often have a great deal of experience of medication, its effects and side-effects. As well as whether or not to take it, there are other choices that they can be given. First, many clients will have first-hand experience of taking numerous different drugs and have views about which has been most effective and had least side-effects for them. From a prescriber's point of view, the chemical action of different drugs in the same class is similar, but their effects and side-effects vary from individual to individual and people often find one more aversive than another. It seems most sensible to ask the person which they prefer, and if they choose the medication it is more likely that they will take it.

Second, most clients will have views about the duration for which medication is given. It is frequently argued that people who experience psychotic disorders must take maintenance medication to prevent their problems reoccurring (Lader, 1995). This is certainly the case for some people: if relapses seriously impede the person's life and destroy the roles and relationships, and if the side-effects of their medication are not too unpleasant or disabling, then they may choose to take medication long term (as is the case with one of the present authors). However, if the side-effects outweigh the benefits then there are other choices. It may well be possible to help a person to identify the first sign of things getting worse and to take drugs when this occurs to prevent relapse (see Birchwood and Tarrier, 1992). For example, one young man was reluctant to take medication because it made it difficult for him to maintain an erection. This seriously jeopardized his relationship with his long-standing girlfriend. On numerous occasions he had been compulsorily admitted following refusal of his maintenance depot medication. It was, however, possible to help him to identify the signs that he might be relapsing and to take medication only when this happened.

Third, the amount of medication that is prescribed is another area where choice is possible. Most people who have ongoing mental health problems have opinions concerning the dosage of medication they take. Professionals tend to regard the appropriate dose of medication as that which minimizes symptoms, whilst the person taking the drugs may have different views. If the dose necessary to minimize symptoms also leaves the person feeling drowsy, lethargic and lacking the energy to do the things that they want to do, then it may well be better for them to take a smaller dose. In our experience, there are many people who prefer to take a dosage that means they have some symptoms but which minimizes side-effects. Such 'sub-optimal' doses of medication may well in fact be optimal in terms of the individual's well-being and day to day functioning. In the context of long term disability, dosages should be judged not in terms of symptom control but in terms of individual preferences, social functioning and facilitating access.

Fourth, a client may also have preferences about the way in which drugs are given: most importantly about the choice between depot and oral medicines. When depot medications first became available they were supposed to be for people who could not reliably take oral preparations – now they are almost invariably the treatment of choice for those deemed to need long term medication. Although depot medication may be preferred by some people, others do not like it. Clearly, the taking of depot medication increases the control that the professional has over the client. The professional can ensure that the client takes the drug in a way that they cannot with oral medicines: the professional has to take it on trust that the client has taken the pills. However, failure to give people this choice can actually decrease the likelihood of their taking medication: over the years we have found that many people are willing to take oral medication but not to take depot injections. For example, two men we worked with had been in and out of hospital for years: they were compulsorily admitted when their distress, disturbance and violent behaviour could not be contained at home, treated with drugs in hospital, discharged when things improved, refused to take injections from the CPN and got more distressed and disturbed until readmitted to hospital. In both cases a switch to oral medication improved the situation. One man was delighted that his request for pills rather than an injection had finally been heard and, in fact, took his pills religiously as the doctor prescribed. Another did not take his pills as prescribed, but he did take the amount that he thought was necessary – and this amount certainly prevented his repeated hospital admissions. What he did was to take a pill every time his head 'felt empty': this on average meant that he was taking half of the prescribed dose. There were arguments amongst the team that he should be put back on a depot injection as he was not 'complying' but, when this was tried, he simply refused his injection – only a timely reversion to oral medication prevented relapse.

Finally, many people have been taking drugs for considerable periods of time and it is simply not known whether they need to continue to take them or not. In general, clinicians adopt a conservative position of recommending continued medication as the best strategy to avert relapse ... even if this advice is not wholly in accord with their own findings. The data from a study by Vaughn and

Leff (1976a) of 128 people with schizophrenia living at home, although designed to look at the effects of a high and low expressed emotion environment, also produced interesting information for the use of maintenance medication. Of those in a low expressed emotion environment, 12% who were on drugs and 15% who were not relapsed in the nine-month period considered. The only reasonable conclusion that can be drawn from these figures is that if a person is living in a low expressed emotion environment then maintenance medication is unnecessary. Drugs did appear to reduce the likelihood of relapse in those living in high expressed emotion environments. Of those who had a high level of contact with their relatives, 53% of those on drugs relapsed as compared with 92% of those not on drugs. In such situations drugs were clearly advantageous. However, if contact with high expressed emotion relatives was reduced below 35 hours per week, the situation was not so clear: 42% of those on drugs relapsed, which means that the majority – 58% – did not.

These results suggest that there may be a lot of people who do not need maintenance medication to prevent relapse and that there are things other than drugs that can be done: change the social environment in which the person is living and/or change the amount of time they spend there. The reality is that, for any given individual who has been taking drugs for some time, we do not know whether they continue to be of benefit. It therefore seems reasonable to allow those who wish to take the risk to try living without the drugs. However, it seems reasonable to assume that such trials are more likely to be successful if they are done in a planned manner, supported by those helping the person. A person may need help and support of a variety of types – emotional, practical, environmental, social, psychological – if they are to maximize their chances of living without medication. Unfortunately, such support is often lacking and the person faces the choice of taking medication, or refusing it and losing the other support that they need. As we have already described, it is not uncommon for a person who refuses their injection to also lose other forms of support such as the fortnightly visit from the CPN who gave them their injection.

We have talked about the many ways in which people who have serious ongoing mental health problems might be given more choice and control over their drugs. It is our opinion that the major problems around medication in mental health services are not the drugs themselves, but issues of power and control: who decides what, how, when and how much medication people take. Most people working in mental health services do not simply take the drugs they are prescribed for physical health problems: most of us would consult a formulary and make our own decisions before taking anything. But we rarely generalize our own actions and experiences to our clients – this is yet another way in which those with mental health problems are too often treated as less than human, people who need to be protected from themselves.

These attitudes may be dysfunctional even within the terms of mental health professionals themselves. Clinicians often talk of 'problems of compliance', 'increasing compliance' – how we can persuade people to do what we think is

best for them. Ironically, there is evidence that by giving people more information and greater choice, 'compliance' can be increased (Day *et al.*, 1995). It is
not our view that the main aim of giving people information and choice is to
ensure that they will do what we tell them to do – our aim must be to enable
disabled people to make choices for themselves, even if we do not approve of
what they are doing. Professionals have formed their opinions on the basis of
information. It this same information is given to clients it seems logical to
assume that many will come to similar conclusions, unless they have additional
information to which professionals rarely have access: what it feels like to take
the drugs involved. This latter information is important – professionals can
learn from their clients.

BEHAVIOURAL THERAPY

There are numerous different behavioural approaches and it is not possible to
consider them all here. We will therefore focus on the two areas that have been
most commonly applied to those with serious ongoing mental health problems:
developing skills and modifying disruptive and difficult behaviour.

A behavioural approach has been used to improve skills in a range of areas
from basic activities of daily living through to social, relationship and work-
related domains. This approach starts with an analysis of the skills involved in
the performance of an activity, whether that activity be filling in an application
form, making a cup of tea, managing one's money or making one's bed. The
second stage involves looking at the person's performance of the task in question and assessing where problems exist. Finally, on the basis of these analyses,
steps are taken to improve the person's performance. There are various strategies that can be adopted in this regard, with a combination of instruction,
prompting, modelling, guided practice and feedback being the most common. In
addition, various forms of contingency management may be used: the contingent presentation or withdrawal of a positive reinforcement or punishment.

Although there is much literature about contingency management and sched-
ules of reinforcement, it is our experience that the achievement of the task is
often intrinsically reinforcing – people feel good about what they have managed
to do – so additional reinforcement is unnecessary. Alternatively, many behaviours elicit their own reinforcing contingencies. For example, if someone does
something positive, it is likely they will automatically elicit positive responses
from others without the need for specific staff intervention. If the behaviour
does not become reinforcing, in and of, itself, or by its naturally occurring
contingencies, then there must be questions about whether it was worth focusing on in the first place: whether it was relevant and meaningful to the person
concerned. The greater challenge is to select the behaviours that are targeted for
development so that they are things that the person wants to achieve (and their
completion will therefore be reinforcing) and change the setting in which the

person functions so that they naturally receive reinforcing recognition for what they have done. This might include working with families and others in the person's social network, to change their view of the individual and recognize their achievements for what they are. For example, one young man very badly wanted to do something useful, but his disabilities were such that no local employers would have him. He did, however, manage with training and help to attend a sheltered workshop. He was delighted with his achievement and went to tell his father, who was unfortunately rather dismissive and asked when he was going to get a proper job. He was extremely dispirited about this and his attendance at the work project stopped – 'What's the point? It's not real work'. Interventions with his family were started to explain to them the nature of their son's disabilities and why, in the light of these, his attendance at the project was so important. He would not return to the previous project but did try another one and, with the encouragement of his father, he has continued to do so. The person providing the reinforcement is often critical – after all, who does value praise from just anyone?

Some of the issues relating to skills training have already been considered in Chapter 2. Whilst it may be possible to teach mechanical skills, any skilled performance involves cognitive components: what to do when, and how, and monitoring and modifying performance in the light of what happens. If a person has cognitive difficulties they may not learn to perform independently the skills we are trying to teach. Indeed, it is often not the skills that have broken down but the effective organization of those skills. If a person has cognitive and emotional disabilities then prompting and encouragement can be vital in enabling them to do things, and are often all that is required to maintain a behaviour. However, they may be required on an ongoing basis. It is probably best to think not about skills training but about establishing and maintaining skilled performance. In this context the ongoing supports that are required to ensure that people can use the skills they have are crucial.

It is important to ensure that a person does not feel belittled or demeaned by the skills training they receive. It is very easy to make a person feel stupid when helping them to do something that any adult would usually expect to do unaided – for example washing and shopping – and clients are often ambivalent about what they have done. The description supplied by one of our clients illustrates this point and also how she came to understand and appreciate her achievements:

> When I first went on the underground I felt great – as if I'd really done something. Then I thought 'What's the big deal, I'm an adult, anyone can go on a train?' Then I realized that while it might not be a big deal for most people I have been in hospital for over 20 years and going on the tube was a big deal for me and I managed it. That's something to be proud of.

A training model with staff as teacher and client as pupil is often not appropriate in a situation where the client's former experiences of education were aversive and unsuccessful. For many people who are seriously disabled by long term mental health problems, school was not pleasant, either because the onset of their problems rendered them isolated, different and unable to excel, or because other social problems pre-dating their mental health difficulties made school an unsuccessful experience. It is easy for skills training to look like a return to an unpleasant educational setting and therefore be aversive, in and of, itself, leaving the person faced, once again, with a powerful teacher who does not really understand their experiences and who is telling them that they are doing things wrong, if not directly then certainly by implication.

The second area where behaviour therapy has been widely used is that of decreasing undesirable behaviours: violence, aggression, sexually inappropriate actions and other disruptive and unacceptable behaviours. As well as instruction and explanation, probably the most commonly used remedy for difficult and aggressive behaviour is 'time out' – but this is a widely misunderstood and misused concept.

In practice, 'time out' often involves a person being taken to a relatively bare/bleak room for a period following the disruptive behaviour. 'Time out' is actually short for 'time out from the possibility of positive reinforcement' and involves removing the person to a place or situation without access to reinforcers. It may be the case that being placed in a 'time out' room is actually reinforcing. For example, a man with whom we worked frequently became disturbed when there were too many people around and if he did not get out of the situation he eventually hit someone – he was then placed in the 'time out' room. This could hardly be considered 'time out from the possibility of positive reinforcement'. Indeed, it might better be understood as positive reinforcement. He got distressed when he was with too many people, when he hit someone he was reinforced by being placed in a less stimulating situation where his distress subsided: the alleviation of distress is reinforcing.

On the other hand, removal to a 'time out' room may not simply be removal from the possibility of reinforcement – it may actually constitute punishment. A young woman had experienced a very deprived and violent childhood that had left her with many problems. She too was intermittently violent to others, especially when she felt misunderstood. When she was violent she was placed in the 'time out' room, where she became even more disturbed and distressed. Her description of the procedure revealed why: 'It's just like when I was a kid – my mother used to shut me under the stairs when I was bad. She shut me there for hours even though I tried and tried to get out. When I got out my hands were often bleeding with scraping at the door. I just can't bear being in that room – it brings it all back.'

When considering the control of violent and aggressive behaviour it is always important to start from a thorough understanding of why the person is behaving as they are. How are they understanding their situation? What is there about their situation that is likely to increase their disturbance and distress? To what extent is their behaviour a direct response to their cognitive difficulties and associated unusual ideas? It is important not only to observe what the person does but to talk to them about how they see things in general, and their violence and disruptive behaviour in particular.

Many people with serious long term mental health problems are understandably frustrated, distressed and angry about what has happened to them, the way they are treated and the ordinary things they cannot have. This in itself can lead to violence. Whilst such behaviour may require short term management strategies to ensure the safety of the person and others, it is vital, in addition, to enable the person to grieve what they have lost and rebuild their life if a permanent solution is to be achieved.

If a person's behaviour is a direct response to their unusual ideas and unshared perceptions, then it is questionable whether a behavioural approach is of any use at all. For example, for over a decade, one man has known that he has been working for the Russians and from time to time they tell him that the staff have set a trap to kill him. When this happens he knows that he has to hit the staff member concerned three times in order to neutralize the trap and avoid death. Manipulating the consequences of this violence is of little use because he is absolutely sure that if he does not hit the staff member he would have died. In this event, and in many other instances of violence and disruptive behaviour, probably the most important thing is to prevent the disruptive behaviour occurring in the first place. This can be achieved in two ways.

First, it can be very important to identify the precursors for that individual and intervene before any violence occurs. For example, in the case of the man described above, before he actually hit staff he became restless, jumping up and down, drumming his fingers on the arm of his chair and hitting his leg. It was observed that this often happened when there were other people around and things going on, and staff surmised that everything was getting too much for him. Therefore, when this restlessness was noted, staff asked him to go and sit somewhere quietly, lie down in his room or go out for a walk with them. This simple intervention reduced his violence by over 75%. The precursors that might be investigated can be aspects of the person's behaviour and demeanour, as with the example given. They may also be environmental events, the behaviour of others or specific frustrations: there are a number of people we know who become irascible and aggressive when they run out of cigarettes for a protracted period.

In addition to, or instead of, identifying precursors of disturbed behaviour, it is often preferable to reinforce alternative desirable behaviours that are incompatible with violence, rather than punish violent and disruptive acts. In order to enable a person to make the best use of their skills it is never enough simply to get rid of unacceptable behaviours – we need to positively help the person to behave in acceptable ways that will enable them to live the lives they want to lead. For example, we worked with one, understandably, very angry young man. He had been in hospital for over a decade and badly wanted to have a job and a home outside. He frequently became angry and aggressive to staff who he saw as preventing him from achieving these things. Instead of focusing on his aggression, we decided to focus on helping him to move towards doing the things that he wanted to do – even if these were some way off. Therefore, he was helped to do jobs within the hospital setting and to start doing cookery and other activities designed to help him to look after himself. At the start of this intervention, many were sceptical and thought he would merely be more dangerous in such settings as a workshop and a kitchen (this was why he had not been referred before). However, with support he was able to do these things and he was never violent whilst engaged in these activities. This experience led to many extensions to his care plan, including activities outside the hospital – visiting hi-fi shops were his favourite – and visits to his parents. Not only did this approach of promoting activities other than violence have the effect of reducing the number of times he hit people, it also increased his own satisfaction because he was able to do things that he valued, and had the spin-off of improving his relationships with staff: instead of only seeing his aggression they were able to engage in positive activities with him.

Whilst behavioural approaches may be useful in some instances, they are probably never sufficient on their own, and can be harmful, because they focus attention on overt behaviour at the expense of the individual's thoughts and feelings. Many people who have serious ongoing mental health problems already feel misunderstood, that no one talks to them, listens to them, or takes what they say seriously. Behavioural approaches, especially those designed to decrease 'difficult' behaviours can reinforce this view – 'difficult' and 'disruptive' behaviours are almost invariably defined not by the person themself but by other people, usually staff. Where they are used, behavioural approaches can probably most usefully be combined with some of the other interventions in an overall package to help the individual to do the things they want in life.

Therapy and disability | 11

The aim of helping someone who has serious ongoing mental health problems is to enable them to have access to roles, relationships, activities and facilities in the community. One such activity or facility is therapy. It is not sufficient simply to offer seriously disabled people therapy; it has to be made accessible to them. In rendering therapy accessible, several considerations are important (Perkins and Dilks, 1992).

At a very basic level, the process of getting to therapy must be addressed. In traditional practice, it is assumed that if a person does not arrive for their therapy session then this has some psychotherapeutic meaning – either in terms of avoidance of difficult issues or a lack of desire for that therapy. When a person fails to attend repeatedly then the therapy is deemed inappropriate and terminated. If this approach were taken in working with people who are seriously disabled by their mental health problems then it is unlikely that many would receive therapy. If people have difficulty in organizing themselves in relation to the world then they often have problems in organizing themselves to get to a therapy session. Enabling a person with such problems to gain access to therapy might involve telephoning them to remind them to come, arranging for someone else to prompt them, organizing transport or taking the therapy to them.

A second access issue revolves around the duration of therapy sessions. It is often not possible to conduct therapy with people who experience serious mental health problems in the traditional '50 minute hour' fashion (Perkins and Dilks, 1992). Such people may not be able to cope with a session of this length: the attentional demands, intensity of interaction or stressful content of a long session may be too great and result in distress or exacerbation of problems. It is important for the therapist to be sensitive to signs that an interaction is exceeding an individual's ability to cope and curtail the session. Warning signs may include the person using diversion in an attempt to remain in control (going to the toilet, going to get a cigarette, changing the subject), an increase in agitation or distress or an increase in the expression of unusual ideas or other cognitive problems.

Along similar lines, as many people experience a fluctuating mental state, it is important to tailor therapy to the constraints that are imposed by the extent of the individual's cognitive and emotional problems at the time. It is important for any therapist to identify what a person can cope with at different times and respond accordingly. For example, when someone is particularly fragile or when their level of disturbance is such that they cannot cope with anything demanding, a brief conversation about something fairly superficial allows the therapist/client relationship to be maintained in a non-threatening way. When the person is able to consider their current experiences, but not able to deal with more distressing issues, then day to day, reality-based problem solving is appropriate. When they are less immediately distressed by cognitive and emotional problems they may be able to address more difficult issues relating to the meaning of their mental health problems, what they have lost as a consequence of their problems and accommodating the reality of their problems into their view of themselves. Often the therapist has the complex task of tracking three separate agendas, adopting in each session the level of interaction that the person can handle at the time and maintaining continuity in each level across time.

The next consideration in therapy is that of developing a trusting relationship. Irrespective of the nature of the therapy employed, its success will, in large part, be dependent upon the quality of the relationship between therapist and client. This relationship must be one in which the client feels that they are valued and understood, able to explore and try out new ideas and activities, and safe to fail without the therapist giving up on them. For this purpose the therapeutic attitudes of empathy, respect and genuineness (as originally defined by Rogers, 1957) are necessary. Patterson and Zderad (1976) have shown that people are more likely to take risks and explore new ideas within a warm, genuine validating and open relationship, whilst Duldt *et al.* (1983) emphasize the importance of a common bond with concern for the client's feelings, needs, worth and responsibility as human beings. However, the particular social disadvantages of people with serious ongoing mental health problems must be taken into consideration.

People with serious ongoing mental health problems have numerous disadvantages which can make it difficult for them to trust other people. Sometimes these relationship difficulties pre-date their mental health problems. Many are disabled not only by their cognitive and emotional problems but also because they have been abused or neglected as children. Many have been in care, experienced sexual abuse, or had parents who were not able to care for them properly because of their own mental health problems and disadvantages. On the other hand, most people in mental health services have experienced many rejections and broken relationships as a consequence of their mental health problems. Many have lost their relationships with family and friends (or these relationships have been distorted beyond recognition), and have lost jobs and social acquaintances. They have also experienced rejection by psychiatric services themselves: numerous short term interventions that were terminated when they 'failed to respond' in the expected manner. Similarly, many have been rejected by a variety of hostels, day facilities and acute psychiatric services.

A history of rejection can make it very difficult to trust new relationships and, quite reasonably, a person may 'test' the relationship: 'I never want to see you again' is often not what they mean. Alternatively, the client may try hard to ensure that the relationship will continue: 'I'm sorry, I did not mean to be rude to you/shout at you/hit you. You are the only person I've ever been able to talk to.' This may make a therapist feel wanted, but is often a sign of the insecurity of the relationship. It is important that a therapist devotes time and attention to the formation of a trusting relationship with a client, and is able to understand 'testing' and 'abuse' as part of the process. This process can be a protracted affair: we have worked with people with whom it has taken over a year to develop a relationship which they feel they can trust and on which they can depend.

In most traditional models it is assumed that therapy is time limited. In relation to someone whose disabilities are ongoing, this can be a grave mistake. Whatever the nature of the therapeutic intervention – whether it be skills training, problem solving or helping the person to adapt to their disabilities and make the most of what they can do – it is often the case that the person's cognitive and emotional problems mean that they require the support of a trusting relationship on a long term basis. Without this they may not sustain day to day activities, deal with new difficulties as they arise or cope with the rejection and stigma that living with serious mental health problems entails.

If a person is unable to structure their internal world, then they can often find lack of structure and direction in the external world particularly threatening and distressing. In a therapeutic context this means that truly non-directive approaches can be particularly difficult. Whilst the therapist must always be sensitive to the needs and wishes of the individual with whom they are working, it is important to structure sessions – to be directive if the person is not able to provide direction for themselves (Bachrach, 1982; Stewart, 1985). As Ekdawi and Conning (1994, p. 81) describe: 'The main objectives should be to attain mastery over internal and external demands and expand the well part, rather than to remove or cure psychopathology'.

Finally, it is important to recognize that many of the skills of psychotherapy are useful outside the context of specific therapy sessions. The basic principles of a counselling approach: careful observation, active listening, skilled questioning, considered interventions and ongoing support form the essential bedrock of many interactions with people who have mental health problems. Specific ongoing therapy can be important, but not for everyone. Most people with serious ongoing mental health problems need a great deal more help and support than therapy alone can provide: a weekly therapy session does not ensure that a person gets enough to eat, has a bath or gets to work. A great many therapeutic strategies and approaches can be useful on an opportunistic basis in the course of other work.

If staff are to be able to take advantage of opportunities for constructive therapeutic encounters with their clients, or to perform specific therapy, a knowledge of the range of interventions available is necessary. However, unless a person has been able to accommodate their mental health problems, and dispel misconceptions and myths about what they mean, the effectiveness of other types of intervention is likely to be decreased.

ADAPTING TO LIFE WITH A DISABILITY

We have already considered the factors contributing to disability and outlined the importance of the way in which a person responds to, or copes with, their problems – their personal reactions to their difficulties (Wing and Freudenberg, 1961; Wing, 1962; Wing and Morris, 1981; Shepherd, 1984). Serious ongoing mental health difficulties are a major life event that profoundly change the course of a person's life. They constitute a bereavement: a loss of the life the person had, or expected to have.

The process of coping with the consequences of serious mental health problems, and the realities of a life with such problems, is difficult not only for the individual, but often for their family and friends as well. However, it is a challenge that such people all too often have to face on their own without anyone to really talk to and share their grief. Diagnoses like 'schizophrenia' often have the quality of a death sentence to the person to whom they are applied, implying that they will be useless, hopeless and unable to do anything ever again. This is compounded by the confusion and fear often associated with the cognitive and emotional problems that have led to this diagnosis (Howe, 1994). It is little wonder that denial and/or hopelessness, with all the disabling consequences that such responses entail, are frequently adopted coping strategies.

People who have serious ongoing mental health problems need to accommodate the things that have happened to them and to adjust to life in a way that minimizes the disabling effects of their difficulties. This process of adaptation involves cognitive and emotional processing that can be made more difficult by their very cognitive and emotional difficulties. Sometimes a person will need assistance in coming to terms with, and adapting to, their problems. It is important to emphasize that mental health workers do not have a monopoly on offering such help, nor are they always in the best position to do so. Support can often be usefully provided by those who have made a similar journey themselves: others who have experienced mental health problems (Lindow, 1993). Whether support is provided by mental health workers or others with similar difficulties, the process of enabling a person to cope involves two main elements.

1. **Grieving.** People need time and opportunity to grieve what they have lost: to express their anger, fear and hopelessness without always being told to 'calm

down', 'pull themselves together' or 'look on the bright side'. This process can take time and is often repetitive, covering the same ground over and over again. Anger, denial, misery and despair are understandable and appropriate responses to the experience of mental health problems in a society that stigmatizes and excludes those with such difficulties. However, it is also important to dispel inaccurate myths about mental health difficulties, and to enable the person to realistically appraise what these mean and do not mean.

2. **Rebuilding: Identifying strengths as well as problems.** In accommodating problems as just one part of the rich tapestry of their lives, the person needs to be able to appreciate their strengths and assets – both those unrelated to their problems and those that they gained as a consequence of their mental health difficulties. People need particular help to maintain a realistic view of what they might expect of themselves: not overambitious as this can lead to failure and demoralization, not too negative and pessimistic as this prevents them reaching their potential.

Achieving these things can take a long time: it is very difficult to value oneself and adjust to a life that so many people in our society (including many clients, their families and friends) regard as worthless. A person needs support if they are to believe in themselves when all their previous conceptions of madness, and those of the people around them, are likely to be condemning them as insane. For many people, any sort of mental distress immediately calls into question the usefulness or validity of any contribution that an individual might make to their family and communities. So help in challenging these preconceptions is vitally important if the handicapping effect of a person's disabilities are to be minimized and they are to regain their self-confidence, make best use of their abilities and live a life that is satisfying.

Clearly, the process of helping a person to achieve these goals must be tailored to their individual needs and problems, but several factors are important. First, in order to feel safe in exploring what can be painful and difficult experiences, an ongoing relationship is necessary: this is not a task for students or temporary staff who will only be available for a short while. Second, the worker must validate the person's emotional responses. Talking about their life, their achievements and ambitions prior to developing problems and how these aspirations have been thwarted by what has happened to them can generate a great deal of misery and anger. It is important that the worker acknowledges and sympathizes with these emotional responses rather than trying to minimize them with phrases like 'It cannot be as bad as all that', 'We haven't really done that to you' or 'We all feel like that sometimes'. Often anger is directed at staff. It is important for the worker not to become defensive about this or argue with the client. It is entirely understandable for the client to become angry with the mental health worker as a representative of the psychiatric system that the person does not want to have to use and which they see as having destroyed their life. Third, helping a person to grieve is not a one-off affair. Processing what has happened can be a lengthy process and the worker should expect to repeatedly listen to what has happened to the person and the emotions associated with it.

If the person does not believe themselves to have mental health problems it is generally not wise to argue with them. Instead, it is possible to talk about the effect of other people **thinking** that they have such difficulties. An exploration of the person's beliefs about what 'mental health problems' are and what they mean is important. Even if the person does not believe that they have such difficulties, this type of discussion can be conducted about mental health problems in general rather than about the individual's specific difficulties. Often someone will not volunteer all their fears about such difficulties, therefore it can be helpful to give explicit permission to raise them. For example, it is possible for the therapist to say such things as 'Some people think that people with mental health problems are violent, or stupid, or lazy ...'. Having understood what a person thinks about mental health difficulties the worker can then proceed to dispel some of the destructive myths they hold. Initially, this can involve an explanation of the nature of the problems, but this should be tailored to the person's preferences and ways of thinking about the world.

Whatever the person's preferred way of understanding mental health problems, it should allow them to build or rebuild their lives and make the best use of their assets. It is important to give the person realistic information about the lives of people with mental health problems. For example, it is important to point out that most people with such difficulties live outside hospital. They do important things: fall in love, have children, get married, run countries, write books, paint, provide services, help others in similar situations, campaign for the rights of those with mental health problems. Contact with campaigning user organizations can provide people with an opportunity to have a valuable role working alongside others in a similar situation to make positive changes.

In helping someone to rebuild their life, it is important to work out what they want to do, what they want to achieve in their lives and how they can make the best of their skills and assets. This process is obviously different for different individuals. For older people it may involve helping them to adapt to retirement and look back on what they have achieved in their lives. A 70-year old man we know had spent some 40 years in hospital and considered his life to have been wasted. It took a long period of time to help him to see that he had fought a considerable fight against the enormous odds of both his mental health problems and decades of hospitalization – a fight that required extraordinary perseverance and bravery. He had also helped a great many other residents in the hospital over the years – making bread in the bakery, assisting in washing and shaving on a ward for elderly people, and helping to cheer up others with whom he lived when they were down.

For people in their middle years who had established an adult life for themselves prior to their problems the task often involves rebuilding a different life. For example, one man lost the home, wife, children and job that he had before his problems began. He moved into a shared house outside hospital, working in a sheltered setting (he still has aspirations towards work in open employment and is quite likely to achieve these), sending money to the wife and children with whom he could no longer have contact and becoming a member of the local Temple.

For people whose entire adult lives have been changed by mental health problems – those who had their first breakdown in their late teens or early 20s – the task is not so much one of rebuilding, but of reformulation and building. Such younger people and their families had many aspirations for what life would hold for them: working, having a home, family, children – an 'ordinary' life. They have to examine how their problems have made achieving these things more difficult and look at the ways in which they may have to change their expectations and circumvent their difficulties to achieve something that is meaningful for them. For example, a man we knew was doing his A levels when his problems began. He had been in care and did not enjoy the support of a family and his problems left him relatively isolated in hospital. His difficulties led him to become interested in philosophy and he wrote a great deal, but he also wanted to have a home of his own and to have a job in which he could pursue his interests. He has been able to achieve these ambitions by living in a supported flat, and although his disabilities have not thus far allowed him to succeed in open employment, he has found voluntary work in a shop specializing in a range of complementary medicines and approaches to health care.

Clearly, it is vital to address the ways in which disabled people come to terms with their experiences in order to live the lives they want to live, but it is not only clients who must make such adaptations. Families, friends and anyone else in the person's social world also have to adapt to disability. Whilst most of the work in this area has related to the parents of a disabled individual, spouses, friends, children and others important to the individual must not be forgotten.

HELPING FAMILIES COPE

In working with people who are seriously socially disabled by their mental health problems it is never possible to treat the individual as an island divorced from their family and social context. The consequences of serious mental health problems are felt more broadly than the individual who experiences them, and if the person is to regain, or preferably maintain, their roles and relationships, then other people who inhabit their life must be considered. Studies have shown that between 50 and 70% of people with a diagnosis of schizophrenia live with their families (Goldman, 1980; Marks *et al.*, 1994), but this varies from place to place. In one Inner London borough it is as low as 14% (Perkins and Arnold, 1994). Many of these people continue to experience cognitive and emotional difficulties and have a high level of social disability which inevitably place psychological, physical and financial demands upon their families. This is compounded by the effects of negative public attitudes towards mental health problems (Hall *et al.*, 1993) and widespread assumptions that the families themselves are to blame (Hatfield, 1989). Not surprisingly, the informal carers of people with serious mental health problems often feel that their needs for information, emotional support and practical help are neglected by services (Shepherd *et al.*, 1994; NSF, 1995). Others in the person's social world may also require information and support if they are to play a useful and positive role in relation to the disabled individual. If communities are to accommodate people with serious mental health problems it is vital that everyone – shopkeepers, employers, workmates, neighbours, people who drink in the pub – understand the realities of serious mental health problems and how they can support those who experience them.

Early approaches to the families of those who experienced serious mental health problems were heavily influenced by the work of theorists like Bateson (Bateson *et al.*, 1956) and Laing (1967), who argued that it was expectations and atmospheres within families that actually caused the problems associated with diagnoses like schizophrenia. With hindsight this perspective had extremely damaging consequences. Many families ceased contact with their disabled offspring because they were told, in one way or another, that it was they who caused their child's problems in the first place. Others have been forced to carry an almost unbearable burden of guilt. In talking with the still distraught mother of a young man who had developed problems 10 years earlier – at the age of 15 – she tearfully asked 'Do you think that if he had been adopted by better people, if I had not been such a bad mother, he would have been all right?'

Recent interest in work with families was pioneered by Brown *et al.* (1958) who noted that people discharged to live with siblings or to lodgings outside the parental family were less likely to relapse than those discharged to live with parents or spouses. Further work revealed that people who returned to live with their mother were less likely to relapse if she went out to work. This led them to hypothesize that relationships within the home, and amount of face to face contact, were of critical importance in predicting relapse (Brown and Birley, 1968). They went on to find that relapse was significantly associated with high levels of 'expressed emotion', indexed by levels of hostility and critical comments on the part of relatives. It appeared that low face to face contact could insulate clients returning to live in homes with high levels of expressed emotion. Vaughn and Leff (1976a, b) continued this work in a controlled study. They found that the risk of relapse of cognitive and emotional difficulties was greatest among those returning to a home environment where levels of critical comments and emotional overinvolvement were high. They noted that relatives behaving in such a way tended to hold inaccurate beliefs about their disabled offspring's behaviour. In particular, such relatives often believed that their child had complete control of their problems and therefore all unusual behaviour was construed as laziness or badness. Alternatively, parents might see their disabled child as completely incapable and in need of continual supervision and help in all areas of life as a small child might.

These findings led to the hypothesis that work with families that included both education about the nature of mental health problems, training in problem solving and more adaptive ways of behaving, might be effective in reducing the level of critical comments and overinvolvement (Leff and Vaughn, 1985). Controlled evaluations of such an approach have demonstrated it to be effective (Leff et al., 1989).

The concept of expressed emotion has been criticized as yet another way of blaming families (Hatfield, 1987). Whilst it does appear to be important to attend to the difficulties of relatives and help them to cope with their child's/spouse's/sibling's problems, later work has suggested that the concept of 'expressed emotion' as such may not be useful. A variety of psychosocial family interventions based on a 'stress-vulnerability' model of serious mental health problems have been developed (Falloon et al., 1984; Tarrier, 1992; Brooker et al., 1994). These approaches are predicated on the assumption that people with such difficulties are particularly vulnerable to social stressors. Interventions with families therefore take the form of education about the nature of disability and vulnerability, stress management and problem solving (as well as decreasing face to face contact time within the family) to decrease the stressors to which the disabled individual is exposed.

Such approaches have been shown to be effective not only to families (Hogarty et al., 1986; Brooker et al., 1994) but also to the disabled family member: reducing cognitive and emotional problems (Falloon et al., 1982, 1985; Tarrier, 1992) and improving social functioning (Falloon et al., 1985; Brooker et al., 1994).

In working with families, several general issues arise. First, our primary loyalty must remain with the disabled individual him/herself. We must be careful to respect their wishes and their confidences. Whilst this may seem obvious it is often easy to respond to the reasonable questions of distraught parents without the permission of the client. For example, we should only contact a person's family with their permission. We must not discuss the client with them without the client's permission. Overall, we must remember that there are often things about our lives that we do nor share with our parents and if we were disabled then there are probably lots of things that we would rather they did not know!

Second, on a related issue, it can cause problems of trust and confidence if the same person is working both with the client individually and with their family. Although it may not always be possible, it is often preferable for different workers to perform these two tasks. This is not only an expressed wish of many individuals and their carers (NSF, 1995), but it also simplifies the worker's responsibilities: attempting to meet the different, even conflicting, needs and wishes of carers and individual whilst respecting confidences and promoting trust is a difficult, if not impossible, task.

Third, we need to think carefully about whether we should see the client and their family together. Whilst there are some models of family intervention that advocate joint working [e.g. Falloon *et al.* (1982) engage the whole family in the task of acquiring behaviourally orientated problem-solving skills as a unit] there is also a case for pragmatism. Just as the client needs space to explore their feelings and experiences on their own, so relatives need their own space to try to understand and cope with their fears and losses.

Fourth, it is vital that we avoid implying, either explicitly or implicitly, that the family are responsible for causing the disabled individual's problems. Although the psychosocial intervention work is based on the assumption that the person's problems do not result from the way relatives have behaved, many families understandably view ideas about 'expressed emotion' as implicitly blaming them (NSF, 1995). It is therefore important that help begins with their needs as they identify them rather than the untailored imposition of a preset programme.

Overall, it is vital that the needs of families and friends are addressed: they constitute a disabled person's social network and as such should be nurtured. In the past, mental health workers have often unwittingly scared off the few social contacts that a disabled person had and neglected those people who provide many of the services formerly offered in large institutions – we must attend to the needs of families and friends, they are the individual's source of social contact and support. We not only do the people with mental health problems a disservice if we scare off the few social contacts that they have but we neglect the people who are increasingly providing the services previously offered by large institutions. The National Schizophrenia Fellowship (NSF, 1988), a relatives' organization, received more than 5000 calls in 1988. Over 3000 were for general advice whilst others were concerned with community care and treatment, family support, accommodation, social services, obtaining benefits, legal advice and hospital care.

Within the various approaches to helping families, a series of areas may be important, many of which parallel the needs of the clients themselves.

Accepting what has happened

Serious mental health problems constitute a bereavement for the family as well as the disabled person. Parents often lose the son/daughter that they once had or expected to have, spouses lose the partner they had, children lose the parent they had. They may also experience guilt, rejection, fear or anger (Kuipers and Bebbington, 1988). Help to grieve these losses, adapt to the possibilities and problems of the future and redefine roles and relationships is often necessary in the same manner as that which we have described for the individual themself.

Education

Relatives, friends and almost all social contacts share the ignorance and myths that surround mental health problems in society. Education about the nature of such problems is as vital for those who have contact with the disabled person as it is for the individual him/herself. Relatives need help to understand the individual's experience and behaviour. Relationships are necessarily tarnished if those around the person incorrectly believe them to be dangerous, lazy and so forth. In such education written material can be important – not only to help the relative to understand what has happened but also to help them to feel less alone.

Sharing

Families often feel isolated and embarrassed by their relatives' behaviour – what will the neighbours think? Enabling them to discuss such unacceptable feelings (disgust, a wish to reject and dissociate themselves and so forth) can be essential if they are not to be destructive. For both the disabled individual and their relatives, one of the most difficult aspects is that mental health problems are often a forced rather than elective choice. The service user faces limited alternatives and relatives may feel guilty when the person is living in less than ideal circumstances (e.g. in bed and breakfast, hostel or hospital accommodation): often they feel they should do more. Promoting contacts with groups and relatives' organizations can enable people to share experiences and feel less alone. Social support is essential for the family as well as the individual. It can reduce the intensity of what can become an all-consuming relationship between the individual and their relative, can provide practical help and can enhance the relatives' self-esteem.

Advice

Family members usually have a strong desire to help their relative who experiences problems but are not always sure what to do for the best (NSF, 1995). Simple problem-solving sessions with the whole family can be helpful: such an approach will be explored further in Chapter 12. These can establish the difficulties and priorities of different members of the family and establish mutually acceptable ways of ameliorating these. Postive contributions can be recognized, problems can be addressed and misunderstandings resolved.

Practical help

Families' needs for practical help are often overlooked. It is easy to focus on the needs of the disabled individual and omit consideration of the family as a whole (Norbeck et al., 1991). For example, the extent to which a family suffers economically often goes unrecognized (Fadden et al., 1987). Sometimes, this might be alleviated by the provision of somewhere for the disabled person to go during the day so that family members can go to work and/or help to ensure that they receive all the benefits to which they are entitled. A study by Creer et al.

(1982) showed that half of relatives had to help their disabled family member with domestic tasks and three-quarters found socially disturbed behaviour problematic. For these, often ageing, people help with the physical demands of care was a priority, as was information about local services and facilities: where to get help when things went wrong and someone to contact when they had difficulties. In short, families need practical information and support in order to continue to support their disabled members.

Monitoring

Families, friends and others in the individual's social world can also have a role in helping to monitor the disabled person's problems and in ensuring that the necessary actions are taken in response to difficulties that arise. In this context, services must respect the opinions of relatives and work with them as partners in ensuring that the individual receives the support they need.

Leaving home

When a young person who is living at home develops serious ongoing mental health problems, relationships are often distorted and it can be difficult for them to grow up and leave home as they would otherwise have done. When a person is not able to cope in the independent manner expected of an adult, it is understandable that parents continue to treat them as a child and are anxious about them branching out on their own. Parents will often need specific support and help to take the risks involved in allowing their child to move away from them and, like anyone else, lead an adult life that may not meet with their approval. Often the most appropriate intervention to make with the family is not to help them to live with the individual with mental health problems but to help them let go and allow their child to move out of the family home.

Advice may also be necessary on reasonable limits on the behaviour of their child. For example, we work with a family whose son had moved out of home but visited them every day for several hours. They felt bad about setting limits on this but also found the constant intrusion unbearable. In negotiations between the child, then 38 years old, and his parents it was agreed that a weekly visit home for Sunday lunch would be acceptable and that, in the interim, the father would go out for a drink with him on Wednesday evenings. This agreement not only benefited the parents, but the ensuing shared activities made the son feel more like the adult he was: going out for a drink with his father has quite a different value to visiting him every day at home.

This latter aspect is important. Too often, relatives get into the habit of visiting their child as they would someone who was sick and in hospital. It is important to ensure both two-way visits and joint activities – like going to the pub – that any parent or child might do. It is also important to discuss how limits will be enforced: for example, parents may need reassurance to deny their child unlimited access to their home.

Providing help and support for the families, friends and acquaintances of people who have serious mental health problems can increase their understanding, well-being and ability to cope. From the client's point of view this can have positive consequences in gaining and maintaining access to ordinary adult roles and relationships as well as improving the quality of these relationships. However, the specific cognitive and emotional difficulties that people with serious ongoing mental health problems experience also require attention. Until the 1980s medication was typically the only intervention offered. Recent developments of specific psychotherapeutic interventions have greatly increased the range of options available.

12 | Coping with specific problems

If a person is to cope with a life that includes serious mental health problems then enhancing their abilities to manage the associated cognitive and emotional difficulties is of utmost importance (Birley, 1995). It is widely recognized that people who have serious mental health difficulties are particularly vulnerable to everyday stresses and problematic life events: these can exacerbate cognitive and emotional problems to an extent that they are unable to cope with day to day life. Helping a person to cope with external stressors and solve problems can therefore be effective in reducing distress and disability, and thereby the need for hospital admission. At its simplest, this involves helping a person to identify those stressors that make their problems worse and decrease their ability to cope, and then enabling them to engage in activities that minimize these negative effects. Helping a person to gain control over their own problems, rather than always having to rely on someone else, is particularly important in developing self-confidence and reducing powerlessness.

SOLVING PROBLEMS

The general principles of problem solving are useful in a wide range of situations and can be used by an individual in relation to particular cognitive or emotional problems, or as a strategy for coping with a variety of challenging situations. Although the process is similar for anyone it must always be adapted to the individual: to fit the situation in which they live and to utilize the coping mechanisms that they have already developed and found effective. Thus, it is a matter of working out what situations a person finds most difficult, or what factors exacerbate their problems, and negotiating a strategy for avoiding that situation and coping with it more effectively. This process involves the following steps.

1. **Identification of the specific problem.** Since it is difficult to deal with lots of problems at the same time, or to solve broad and general difficulties, it is important to focus on one specific difficulty at a time. This is not always

easy, skilled questioning and active listening will be necessary to move from such vague complaints as 'I hate my flat' to more specific problems: 'My neighbours make a noise in the middle of the night', 'I'm scared of the teenagers who live downstairs' or 'It's too cold here'. There will be times when a long list of problems is generated and it is necessary to prioritize those that are most distressing.

2. **Identifying possible courses of action.** Again, the person may need help to identify the action they could take to overcome the problem. This might involve discussing the ways they normally cope, what is most effective and what else could be tried. It is important not to be selective at this stage but to enable them to recognize the range of options that are not only available to them but which they already know about. For example, in relation to noisy neighbours 'I could talk to my neighbours about the noise', 'I could call the police', 'I could complain to the council', 'I could buy some ear plugs' or 'I could ask for a transfer'. It may be appropriate to draw their attention to possible courses of action which they have not thought of, or it might be necessary to look into further possibilities through research outside the session.

3. **Selecting a course of action.** Every possible course of action should be considered in terms of its advantages and disadvantages. It is essential that the mental health worker does not simply prescribe a course of action but instead systematically helps the person to consider the pros and cons of all possible options. In this way the client can develop a generalizable strategy for solving difficulties, not simply a specific solution to the immediate problem. It can also be helpful for the person to consult others and obtain their views: most people get the opinions of their family, friends or colleagues when they have difficulties. Eventually, a decision must be made about the most appropriate action. This may not involve selecting just one course, but deciding on a series of actions, or on alternative measures if the first course does not have the desired effect. For example, the first step may be to approach noisy neighbours and ask them to be quieter. If this is ineffective, the police may be called and, as a last resort, the person could request a housing transfer.

4. **Action.** In taking action, a clear plan must be laid out. This should be based upon realistic steps, and importantly it will involve support and encouragement. A person may find it helpful to rehearse what they will do and when they will do it, for example, when to approach the neighbours and what to say to them. At times, regular meetings to monitor progress will be sufficient, but in other situations it might be necessary to enlist the help of other people: it may be easier to go with a friend to confront the neighbours about their noise. Things do not always work out correctly first time. It will most probably take time and a number of attempts, if not a change in plans, before

the desired results are effected. An important part of the ongoing support is the evaluation of the effects of the actions taken and the modification of plans in the light of experience.

This type of guided practice can not only develop solutions to particular problems, but also offers a strategy for approaching new ones. However, it clearly imposes considerable cognitive demands which can be particularly problematic for someone with the cognitive difficulties associated with serious mental health problems. Sometimes problem-solving interventions are seen as time limited: teaching the person a series of techniques that they can then go on and use on their own, or helping a person cope with a particular problem with support only for as long as the difficulty lasts. However, when a person has cognitive difficulties the assistance of someone else as a 'prosthetic aid' to resolving difficulties as they arise may be necessary for a protracted period, if not indefinitely. For example, one woman had been in and out of hospital several times per year for over 10 years before she was finally unable to return to her flat and became a long-stay patient. It rapidly became obvious that every time a problem arose – difficulties with her son, an argument with friends, the television breaking down, a bill arriving – she could not cope, her symptoms became worse and she had to return to hospital. We began working with her nearly eight years ago in order to help her to manage such difficulties more effectively. A problem-solving approach was adopted every time a difficulty (however small) arose. Gradually her problem-solving skills improved. She was able to leave hospital and for three years she lived in a supported setting, but her ambition remained to have a place of her own. After a year of making no demands on the housing support team she was able to achieve this ambition: she has been living in her own flat for over a year. Throughout this period she has seen a mental health worker at least weekly, and the primary component of this input has been to help her to use her problem-solving skills. As yet, she has never been able to use these unaided. Every time a problem arises her cognitive problems get worse and she becomes distressed, but with ongoing support she is able to employ a problem-solving strategy to resolve difficulties without jeopardizing her community tenure. It is important to emphasize that the mental health worker does not solve problems for her but assists her in resolving them herself.

Thus far we have talked only about a problem-solving approach in relation to external events, and there is evidence that people with serious mental health problems are well able to appreciate the links between these external stressors and a worsening of their cognitive and emotional problems (Wing, 1983). However, there are other areas in which problem solving can be useful. Although the woman described above has not had to return to hospital, she has had to contend with worsening of her problems (hearing voices, difficulty in organizing her thoughts and beliefs that her room has been bugged): a problem-solving strategy has been effective with these as well. Problem-solving approaches are useful both in relation to external events that exacerbate cognitive and emotional problems and in dealing with these problems themselves.

MANAGING SYMPTOMS

Most people do develop strategies for coping with the distressing cognitive and emotional problems they experience (Dittman, 1990), usually on a trial and error basis, exploring what works. Whilst these are not always successful, there is evidence that the systematic teaching of a variety of strategies can be helpful (Tarrier, 1992). As different individuals find different strategies useful, it is best to explore with the individual the precise nature of their problems, the extent to which they are distressing or interfere with other activities, the strategies that they have evolved to cope themselves and the effectiveness of these. It is important to recognize that not all cognitive difficulties are distressing or disabling: many people are not upset by, for example, hearing voices, and do not find their unusual beliefs aversive. There is nothing to be gained from trying to change something that is neither distressing nor disabling for the sake of 'normality'.

Having identified problems and existing coping strategies, the next step is to look for clues concerning alternative coping strategies that might be more effective. This can usefully be done by looking at the natural variability in the problems identified. Unusual beliefs and other cognitive problems are not fixed or stable and the way in which they change across time and situations can give clues about what might exacerbate and ameliorate them: make them better or worse. It is possible to talk this through with a person, asking them to think over that last day and say when they were better and when they were worse. It may be possible for a person to keep records to get this information: noting when their problems are worse/better and what they were doing, or what was happening, at the time.

Although the most useful information will come from the person themself – it is, after all, very difficult for others to see if a person has a particular internal experience or idea – there may be behavioural correlates of these that allow mental health workers, relatives or friends to observe what is going on. With all the information collected it is possible for client and mental health worker to set up hypotheses about strategies that might be effective. For example, if the person's problems are worse when there are a lot of people around it may be useful for them to take themself to a quieter situation if things get bad. Alternatively, if the problems always occur when the person has nothing to do it may be possible to arrange for them to have access to activities to decrease the distress caused by their problems. Different strategies are likely to be appropriate for different individuals. Among our own clients, these include: going for a walk, going to lie down, asking for 'as-required' medication, listening to music, watching the television, talking to someone, reading, repeatedly telling the voices to 'go away' in some way and asking them to come back at a more convenient time, writing, and singing. This list is not exhaustive and it should not be taken as a recipe that can simply be given to people. It represents 'detective' work on the part of clients to find things that worked for them. Often people use a variety of different strategies in different situations and for different problems, but in every case they must make sense to the individual themself and not simply represent the prescriptions of the worker.

Once strategies have been identified, it is necessary to work out how they will be used and help the person to use them. For example, it is necessary to work out how reading matter can be made available to the person (a magazine in her handbag), where they can get 'as-required' medication and so on. In order to use the strategies to maximum effect, the person not only needs to work out how to use the strategy but also when to use it. They have to monitor their problems and note when they **begin** to get worse: it is usually more effective to employ a coping strategy when difficulties are beginning rather than when they are already at their worst. Various prompts may be useful to remind the person to use coping strategies. These might include written notes/instructions and reminders from other people. Finally, it is important to evaluate the effectiveness and acceptability of the strategies with the person concerned, and adapt them, add to them or seek alternatives as appropriate.

Serious mental health problems often leave a person feeling that they have no control over their internal thoughts and feelings, let alone over external events. This is a terrifying experience that can destroy any sense of personal agency and integrity. Anything that can increase a person's control over their own life and experience is extremely important. Problem solving in relation to external and internal difficulties is one approach, but there are others. In particular, people can also gain control via monitoring their own cognitive and emotional problems, minimizing the likelihood of relapse and, as a last resort, determining what will happen if a crisis does occur.

MONITORING RELAPSE

Many people with serious long term mental health problems experience periodic crises: reducing and coping with these is important for two major reasons. First, every relapse increases the probability of future crises and tend to result in increased social disability (Hogarty *et al.*, 1986). Second, repeated crises leave people feeling out of control over their lives: they are reluctant to plan for the future, even the relatively immediate future, because they never know whether they will be able to do what they intend to do. Strauss *et al.* (1989), on the basis of people's own accounts of their problems, describe the demoralization that can arise as a direct result of repeated exacerbation of cognitive and emotional problems. He cites some of the social and psychological situations that lead to withdrawal, apathy, avoidance and hopelessness.

- Fear of relapse may lead to a person giving up activities which they previously enjoyed but which they associate with intensified cognitive difficulties.
- The loss of hope and self-esteem may result from repeated admissions which lead to the breakdown of employment, as well as family and social contacts.
- Apathy and withdrawal may be the only means a person knows of avoiding a recurrence of embarrassing behaviour.
- A person may lack any identity other than that of 'patient': this can become the only framework they have for relating to others and getting help, and they are understandably fearful of giving it up.
- A person may feel pressure to withdraw and give up through feelings of guilt about behaviour when they were in crisis, or at being unable to perform in roles they had previously enjoyed.

Fluctuating cognitive and emotional problems are not only distressing for the person who experiences them but also for those around them, making the person appear unreliable and unpredictable. For these reasons, interest over recent years has focused on techniques for helping to reduce the risk of crises occurring and minimizing their severity and the disturbance which they cause. Techniques for preventing and minimizing relapse have been pioneered by Birchwood *et al.* (1992) using a broadly cognitive–behavioural model.

This approach involves a series of elements. Probably the most important component is identifying the individual's 'relapse signature': that singular pattern of experiences that heralds a crisis. Each person's experiences will be different, so a thoroughly individualized approach is required. There are often two primary stages: dysphoria (including anxiety and restlessness) followed by early cognitive problems such as suspiciousness and misinterpretations. In identifying the person's 'relapse signature' their own account is the most useful, but signs can also be observed by relatives, friends and other carers. In helping a person to identify and monitor the early signs of an impending crisis, it is important to use their own words and descriptions. Although a mental health worker may interpret a specific experience, such as 'I get fidgety' in psychiatric terms (such as restlessness), it is best to use the person's own description in helping them to monitor themselves.

Having outlined the components of the individual's 'relapse signature', the next step is to help them develop ways of monitoring their problems. Sometimes this can involve written records. For example, one man experienced infrasound waves disrupting his thoughts most of the time. Generally they were very strong first thing in the morning but became weaker by about 9–10 am, allowing him to go about his business of the day with little interruption. However, when he began to relapse they did not subside until later in the day. He was well able to calibrate the strength of the infrasound on a 10-point scale and, given the pattern of his relapses, he monitored himself at midday each day. If the infrasound at this time was less than five on his scale then things were all right, if it got above this level then things were not so good and he needed to take action.

Sometimes people do not find such monitoring very easy and can benefit from assistance. One woman noted that one of the first indicators that things were getting worse for her was failing to sleep at night. She was not able to keep written records about her sleep but she was able to report on it verbally. Therefore, a brief telephone call on alternate days was used to check how she had been sleeping. It is important not only to gain information about the pattern of a person's crises but also to gain an idea of time scale. In the example given above, the woman's sleeplessness typically lasted 3–4 days before other more serious problems emerged. Therefore, she was called every two days to ensure that she was able to act in the early stages before things got too bad. If her sleepless phase had lasted for a longer period then such frequent checking may not have been necessary. The early identification of an impending crisis is important not only to prevent further deterioration but also to enable a person to remain in control of what is happening to them.

Once a person's 'relapse signature' has been identified and a monitoring system established, a series of strategies and interventions can be designed to reduce the likelihood and severity of the crisis. On the one hand, there may be things that the individual can do to identify any stressors that might be exacerbating the problems and take steps to reduce these. The problem-solving type of approach already discussed can be useful in this regard. On the other hand, a person may be encouraged to seek help. Such help could take any form that is deemed effective: increased support at home, day care, admission or increased medication.

This process was particularly effective with one of our clients. A woman, with a diagnosis of schizo-affective disorder, had a typical 'revolving door' pattern of service use: receiving very little input between admissions of an increasing duration and frequency. Typically, her admissions were compulsory and associated with extreme self-neglect, self-harm and suicide attempts. When we began to work with her it became clear that she was well aware when things were starting to go wrong and would have been happy to accept help in the early stages of her crises had such help been readily available at the time when it was needed. Together, we worked out her 'relapse signature' and what she should do at each stage (see Table 12.1). In her experience there were four stages – our plan can be seen in the table. It is important to emphasize that everyone else involved was primed to respond as we indicated. The ward were involved so that her requests for admission and assistance would be treated with the gravity they deserved and they agreed to tell her friends where she was (she was reluctant to let them down). We discussed her request for someone to accompany her in the bus or taxi with two of her friends, both of whom agreed to help. We supplied her with a £5 sealed in an envelope as the fare for the taxi could be a problem.

Table 12.1 'Relapse signature' and plan of action for each stage for a patient with a schizo-affective disorder

Stage 1	Stage 2	Stage 3	Stage 4
Unable to sleep at night Lethargic – not wanting to do things Irritable with friends Often occurs after a period of doing a great deal or when problems have arisen	Voices whispering in my head The ground feels spongy Finding it hard to go out Pain in the bottom of my neck	Voices very loud Cannot go out Cannot eat anything	Voices and bubbles intolerable Little green and red men to the left Wanting to harm yourself – cannot see any point in carrying on Thoughts racing all over the place Too scared to get out of bed
Take it easy Cancel some social engagements (don't go out more than two nights per week) Tell friends that you are not feeling so good and need a rest for a few days Make a note of problems to discuss with Rachel on her next visit	Take a bus to the ward, explain the situation and ask to be admitted for a while If necessary call a friend and ask her to go with you Call Rachel when you get there Ask staff to call and cancel any dates with friends that you have	Call a taxi to take you to hospital Use the £5 note in the envelope at the bottom of your bag to pay for it If necessary ask a friend to go in the taxi with you Ask staff to call Rachel and cancel any dates with friends	Call the ward and ask them to come and get you immediately
If no better after a week follow instructions for Stage 2	If unable to get to hospital by bus follow instructions for Stage 3	If unable to get to hospital by taxi follow instructions for Stage 4	

This type of approach can be useful wherever a person has fluctuating cognitive and emotional problems, but can be particularly important if a person does not want to take maintenance medication: it can be used as a framework for offering the person positive and constructive support in their attempts to live without drugs. Instead of entering a destructive battle over medication, this type of 'relapse-prevention' strategy can be used to enable people who want to try living without long term neuroleptics to do so, whilst at the same time minimizing disabling crises (Birchwood *et al.*, 1992).

Throughout this type of monitoring and relapse prevention/planning approach, it is important to emphasize that catastrophizing should be minimized. The aim is to enhance self-control rather than to generate panic and alarm: to prevent a full-blown crisis by catching and aborting it at an early stage, and so decrease distress and disability. However, there are other interventions that can be used more directly to reduce cognitive problems.

REDUCING SYMPTOMS

Although medication is the most commonly used intervention for alleviating serious cognitive problems it is not a popular treatment. A large number of people find its side-effects distressing and its effectiveness is limited (Lader, 1995). This situation has prompted the development of other ways of addressing unusual and distressing beliefs and perceptions, such as hearing voices.

In relation to hearing voices, we have already described approaches for enhancing a person's coping strategies (Tarrier *et al.*, 1988). However, self-help can be at least as important as professional intervention. Often it is not the hearing of voices in, and of, itself that is problematic, but the fear and distress that they can engender as well as a sense of being out of control: having to do what they say. Such fear can be alleviated by contact with others who have similar experiences. In a self-help context, people who hear voices can have a frank and open interchange: assured of the understanding that can never be forthcoming from those who do not share their experiences (Romme *et al.*, 1992). This can reduce stigma, isolation and fear, and can also increase control through sharing ideas with other experts (people who also hear voices): it has become evident that people can develop relationships with their voices that allow amicable cohabitation. For example, one woman found that if she set aside a particular time each day to talk to her voices then they did not interrupt her while she slept or worked. Some voices are nice and some remain nasty: a person may not like their voices but they can learn to live with them and modify the influence they have over their lives.

Some people find mechanical aids, such as ear plugs and headphone music, useful in reducing their voices. Done *et al.* (1986) found that wearing an ear plug in the dominant ear decreased frequency and volume of auditory hallucinations, although why this worked was unclear. Morley (1987) and Hustig *et al.* (1990) found that a personal stereo could decrease the extent to which voices impinged on what a person was trying to do: some people found music most effective, whilst others preferred speech or 'white noise', and the preferred volume varied. It is also worth noting that, whilst beneficial for some people, use of a personal stereo worsened the voices of others.

There has been an increased interest in the thinking and reasoning styles associated with strange and unusual beliefs (Huq *et al.*, 1988; Bentall *et al.*, 1989). This has led to the development of a variety of cognitive approaches to address them (Chadwick and Lowe, 1990). Such approaches essentially involve three stages. First, talking to the person about their beliefs to identify those that are most distressing or disturbing. These will then become the target of intervention.   Second, thoroughly exploring the beliefs by gathering information about their precise nature and the evidence that the person uses to support them (for example, 'I know I am a German because my mother had fair hair, and Germans have fair hair, and when I was a child I didn't have ordinary measles I had German measles'.). People use a variety of types of evidence to support any belief and unusual beliefs are no different. Some will be more central than others, so the person is asked to rank the importance of the evidence in supporting the belief that they hold. Third, encouraging the person to view their belief as just one way of interpreting the evidence. There are always many different ways of understanding the same things and the person is asked to identify some of these alternatives. The alternative explanations for each piece of evidence are explored, thus challenging the belief itself. For example, it may be important to look at other nationalities in which fair hair is common and the range of different nationals who contract German measles.

Throughout this process of exploring a person's beliefs and the supporting evidence, it is essential that confrontation is avoided. We have discussed the way in which denying the reality of a client can prevent the formation of an effective relationship (Perkins and Dilks, 1992) and impede other areas of performance. If the client feels that they are being told that their belief is untrue then this can have the paradoxical effect of causing them to justify it with further evidence, and thus strengthening rather than weakening their certainty. Ekdawi and Conning (1994) cite the example of a young man whose self-confidence and functioning were eroded because of constant challenges to a firmly-held unusual belief. When such negative attention ceased, and staff accepted his interpretation of events, his mood lifted, and his functioning and self-esteem improved sufficiently to allow him to move into independent accommodation.

Cognitive approaches directed towards helping people with serious mental health problems have attracted a great deal of interest. On an individual client basis they have proved effective, but large-scale studies are not yet available. Probably the most important contribution of these and other psychotherapeutic approaches is that they take seriously the concerns, experiences and expertise of people with serious cognitive and emotional problems, rather than dismissing them as mere symptoms of illness.

Overview: Talking, listening and hearing

Any intervention to help people with serious ongoing mental health problems should be aimed towards enabling them to gain control over their problems and lives. Listening to clients, believing what they say and helping them to do the things they want in life are of the essence. This may not sound radical but, whilst there are encouraging developments, the sad reality remains that, for most people with serious cognitive and emotional problems, medication is the primary help they are offered.

Listening to clients, hearing what they say and acting upon it essentially involves according them power and control and this involves decreasing the power of professionals to determine what is best for them. Giving service users power to say what happens to them takes away that power from mental health workers. It is very difficult to stand by and help someone to do something that we believe to be potentially harmful, and there are some instances when mental health legislation forbids this. However, if we are really to serve our clients well – helping them to gain control over their own lives and do the things they want to do – then we must be prepared to help them do this. Just as different mental health workers have different ideas about what is best, so clients' views will sometimes differ from our own.

This does not remove the role of professional expertise, it merely changes it. It is the way in which that expertise is made available to clients, and who controls how that expertise is used, that is important. Anyone needs to be given information, advice and help if they are to make informed choices: no one can be an expert in everything. But few of us like to be dictated to by others. We need to change the role of expertise from that of telling people what to do to that of advising, informing and supporting them to make their own decisions and realize them. Recent psychotherapeutic developments increase the range of options that mental health workers can offer, but they must not be prescribed like pills. Further, it is important for all mental health workers to recognize the expertise that they often lack: that expertise endowed by the personal experience of cognitive and emotional problems. Many future developments are likely to further capitalize on the expertise and wisdom of such experience (Chamberlin, 1977; Lindlow, 1993; Deegan, 1993).

There are numerous ways in which everyday practice can be changed to shift the balance of power and allow people greater control. On a large scale, one particularly graphic example of such a shift can be found in Portland, Oregon, where a consumer-run intensive case management team employed a psychiatrist: the psychiatrist was working for the people with mental health problems who run the service (Perkins, 1993). At the other end of the scale, any mental health worker can, despite all resource constraints, listen to the people with whom they work, believe what they say, help them to do the things that they want to do and increase the extent to which they have control over their lives.

PART FIVE

Some Challenges for the Future

Introduction

Throughout this book we have outlined many challenges that face those who provide services for people who experience serious ongoing mental health problems. Probably the most important task is to move away from the position of patients using **our** services, towards one in which we are **serving** the people who need support. This involves moving a position in which **we** know what is best for **our** clients to one in which clients determine what they want to achieve and we place our expertise at their disposal.

We have argued that those people whom we serve have the same needs as anyone else, but may need additional help in meeting these needs because of their disabilities – disabilities that result both from cognitive and emotional difficulties and stigma and social disadvantages that, within our society, are consequent upon the experience of mental health problems. Most importantly, we must make our services both accessible to our clients and acceptable to them. Instead of focusing upon compulsion – new ways of making people accept help – we should consider primarily how we can render our services attractive so that people want to use them. Only a part of rendering services acceptable can be achieved through changes in the bricks and mortar: the most important factor is our relationships with clients. If we can really treat those who we serve with dignity and respect, if we can really listen to their concerns and wishes and act upon them, if we can provide support without belittling and infantilizing them, then we can go a long way towards making services appropriate, improving clients' experience of them and therefore increasing the likelihood that they will use them when they need them.

Within this context there are several groups of people in relation to whom mental health services fare particularly badly, and it is to these clients that the first two chapters in this section will be devoted. First, there are those people who, in addition to the stigma and exclusion associated with mental health problems, also have to face oppression because they are black, female, lesbian or gay. Second, there are those whose problems do not fit neatly with our expectations and who do not use mental health services in the manner intended. Some of these people are elderly and have needs that span adult mental health services and services for older people. Others have learning disabilities or physical/sensory disabilities in addition to their mental health problems, others have degenerative diseases like Huntington's chorea or the cognitive deficits associated with Korsakoff's psychosis or pre-senile dementia. Such people are often the subject of 'boundary disputes' between the different services that might meet their needs. There are no absolute rules in such conflicts: decisions about who might best provide the support they need depends upon the individual and these may change over time. We have worked with a young woman who was diagnosed as having schizophrenia in addition to pre-lingual deafness and learning disabilities. Initially, she was provided with care in a service designed for people with pre-lingual deafness, but her disturbed and disruptive behaviour could not be accommodated within such services: she was often frustrated because she could not meet the demands of the situation as a consequence of her learning disabilities and she found a signing environment overstimulating because of the cognitive deficits associated with her mental health problems. She was transferred to a mental health service for people with challenging behaviours and initially did well: her disturbed behaviour decreased and in the highly structured and supervised setting that this placement afforded she was able to engage in a variety of work and social activities. However, she remained relatively socially isolated. Other residents, in an attempt to be kindly, treated her as a backward child and did things for her. Most importantly, she was extremely sexually and financially vulnerable: when others were taking advantage of her she understandably became very distressed and began to harm herself. Within a mixed mental health unit she could only be rendered safe by having a member of staff with her at all times (day and night). Clearly, a single sex unit may have been able to meet her needs, but no such facility was available. She was eventually placed in a community for people with learning disabilities and in this context has flourished. She has many friends, is able to engage in an enormous range of activities that are conducted at a pace which she can handle. She also has a boyfriend who visits and stays with her every weekend and showers her with presents. At last, she seems to be happy and all her former disturbed behaviour has ceased.

Whilst issues of which service might best be in a position to support people whose multiple needs span the expertise and resources available in different services, probably the biggest challenge to community care comes from a group of people who have a diagnosis of 'personality disorder' in addition to, or instead of, mental health problems and who often behave in ways that services do not like. It is this group of people who will form the subject matter of the second chapter in this section. We will consider the challenge that they pose to services and ways in which we might set about meeting this challenge. It is our contention that meeting the challenges posed by those who currently fail to 'fit in' with that which is offered is likely to render services more appropriate and acceptable to all who require them.

Finally, we will move on to consider some of the changes in direction that will be necessary over the next decade. Many services for people with long term mental health problems have been developed in the context of closing large mental hospitals. When these large mental hospitals have been closed the problems for future generations will be different: people who develop serious cognitive and emotional problems will no longer enter long-stay hospital wards from which they must be resettled, as these wards will not exist. Services will need a change in focus to enable people to retain homes and roles in the community from the start.

Whose community is it anyway? Doubly disadvantaged groups

13

People who experience serious ongoing mental health problems are typically marginalized and excluded from the communities in which they live. In former times, this exclusion was achieved through prolonged incarceration in distant mental institutions. In an era of care in the community it tends to take more subtle forms. The majority of those who would formerly have been institutionalized today live 'in the community'. However, it remains rare for this physical presence in communities to be associated with a genuine integration into, and acceptance by, the communities in which they reside: people may be **in** 'the community', but they are rarely a valued and respected part of it. Many seriously disabled people living outside hospital remain extremely socially isolated (Beels *et al.*, 1984; Warden *et al.*, 1990) and those contacts which they do have tend to be in segregated settings inhabited only by others with mental health problems: day centres, sheltered workshops, drop-ins and so forth. Too often the role of 'mental patient' remains in the ascendancy and obscures all other facets of the person.

The stigma, exclusion and ensuing isolation of a person with serious mental health problems cannot be underestimated. For those who have the additional disadvantages that are a consequence of being a part of other oppressed groups, the position is dramatically worse. A person who is black, female, lesbian, gay, working class, old, physically disabled as well as having serious mental health problems is doubly, or triply or quadruply disadvantaged. We will focus primarily on blacks, women, lesbians and gays, but many similar arguments can be made in relation to age, class and physical disability.

At the outset it is important to emphasize that in considering the experiences of these diverse groups together we are not suggesting that the nature of the oppression experienced by each is the same. The experience of someone who is black is quite different from that of someone who is lesbian and that of a black

lesbian is different again. The specific disadvantages of each group are important and have been considered at length elsewhere (see Chesler, 1972; Mowbray
et al., 1985; Perkins, 1991a, 1992a, 1995; Harrison *et al.*, 1988; Francis *et al.*,
1989; Moodley and Perkins, 1991; Fernando, 1991; King *et al.*, 1994; Perkins
and Fisher, 1995a). However, at both a practical and a conceptual level, there
are common themes in relation to 'community care' that can usefully be
explored and it is towards these that we will direct our attention.

THE RELATIVE NATURE OF SOCIAL DISABILITY

As we have seen, someone who experiences serious ongoing mental health
problems is socially disabled in that they are unable to perform to the standards
that are expected of them. People require long term support not because of their
cognitive and emotional problems *per se*, but because of the social impact of
these and the social disadvantages that the experience of mental health problems
entails. However, social disability cannot be considered in a vacuum – a person
can only be considered disabled in relation to a specific social context or group.

The social world in which all social groups must live is one that is defined by
white, heterosexual men (see Kitzinger and Perkins, 1993; Perkins, 1995).
Within such a world the sexist, racist and heterosexist assumptions that abound
are inherently oppressive for women, blacks, lesbians and gay men. People
from oppressed groups are marginalized and excluded because of their failure to
meet white, heterosexual male norms. But there are communities of oppressed
people – lesbian communities, gay communities, African Caribbean communities, Asian communities – with their own cultures, beliefs, institutions and
prescriptions.

Many oppressed groups have argued how blacks, lesbians, gays and women
have been defined as mad because they contravene the norms set by a white
heterosexual male society (see Chesler, 1972; Kitzinger and Perkins, 1993;
Fernando, 1991).

Feminist theory has always pointed out that some of what is conventionally
labelled as madness is in fact ordinary behaviour for women. In 1972, Phyllis
Chesler argued that madness in women is a direct result of male-defined notions
of femininity:

> There is a double standard of mental health – one for men, the other for
> women – existing among clinicians ... For a woman to be healthy, she
> must 'adjust' to accept the behavioural norms of her sex – passivity,
> acquiescence, self-sacrifice, and lack of ambition – even though these
> kinds of 'loser' behaviours are generally regarded as socially undesirable
> (i.e. non-masculine).

Chesler, 1972

Similarly, Louise Pembroke, former chair of the user organization 'Survivors Speak Out' describes how she

... discovered at an early age that a woman's worth is gauged by her appearance; expressions of anger and assertion are not easily tolerated; that my low place in society's pecking order has nothing to do with me but is connected to the maintenance of a hierarchy based on white male dominance.

Pembroke, 1991

We have seen, within services in which we have worked, women deemed to have 'improved' because they have put on make-up, done their hair and dressed in a feminine manner (Johnstone, 1989). We have seen that which passes for a 'women's group' devote inordinate amounts of time to make-up and nail painting (Perkins, 1991a). We have heard 'living at the Greenham Common peace camp' listed as one of the features of a woman's psychopathology. In short, women may be labelled as mad because they deviate from male prescriptions of female behaviour in a world that legitimizes women's second-class status and urges us to view our identity in terms of our success as wives, mothers and sexual companions.

In a similar fashion, lesbianism and male homosexuality have long been deemed pathological. For example, Kronemeyer (1980, p. 7) described homosexuality as:

... a symptom of neurosis and of a grievous personality disorder. It is an outgrowth of deeply rooted emotional deprivations and disturbances that had their origins in infancy. It is manifested, all too often, by compulsive destructive behaviour that is the very antithesis of fulfilment and happiness. Buried under the 'gay' exterior of the homosexual is the hurt and rage that crippled his or her capacity for true maturation, for healthy growth and love.

It continues to be the case that two of the UK's leading psychoanalytic training institutes will not train 'out' lesbian and gay therapists, and lesbianism and male homosexuality are used as indices of disturbance (Kitzinger, 1990). Further, the World Federation for Mental Health (1992) in its Human Rights Bill for Hospitalised Mental Patients includes the right:

To have suitable opportunities for interaction with members of the opposite sex.

It is not only lesbians who might want respite from having to interact with men. Many heterosexual women, as well as lesbians, have campaigned for single-sex facilities because of the harassment and abuse they have experienced in mental health settings (Gorman, 1992). We have heard several male professionals argue that mixed-sex facilities are 'normal': it is normal for women to live with men. Not only does this deny the reality and experience of many women, but it is also a gross misrepresentation of the situation of most women: most of us do **not** live with male strangers who are not of our choosing. A woman with serious long term mental health problems living in a shared community supported house told us (Perkins, 1995):

I'm not safe out there. I'm not safe in here. Where are you safe?

Another said:

We need protection. Protection from being attacked. And protection from always being nagged for cigarettes, lights, and sex. The men threaten to hit you if you don't give them what they want.

In one continuing community care service, the most common reason given by women for refusing sheltered accommodation was that they would have to live with men (Repper and Perkins, 1995). We are pleased to be able to recount that, since this came to light, women-only accommodation has been made available in this service.

Often, heterosexism takes relatively subtle forms but it is no less oppressive for this (Falco, 1991). It is not uncommon for mental health professionals to reassure clients who think they might be lesbian or gay that they are not. This is particularly common in work with younger lesbians and gay men, and the argument can take many forms: you are not lesbian because you have had relationships with men in the past, or because you have never had a relationship with a man (so how could you know?), or because you have had a bad relationship with a man (you must not condemn all men on the basis of one rotten apple), or because you were abused as a child, or because everyone of your age has crushes on women and they do not mean a thing ...

Alternatively, assumptions within services that everyone is heterosexual (that reflect those prevailing in society at large) mean that the possibility that a person is lesbian/gay is simply never explored or recognized. Given the extent of anti-lesbian/gay attitudes, most clients deem it sensible not to reveal their identity. A further heterosexist attitude in services is one that applies equally to blacks, women and members of other oppressed groups. It is an approach which says that being black, or lesbian, or gay, or female, simply does not matter: 'We treat everyone the same here, irrespective of the colour of their skin, sex, or sexuality', 'What you do in bed is your own business', 'The fact that you are black or female (or both) is irrelevant'. This apparently liberal attitude is extremely oppressive as it ignores the fact that being black, or lesbian, or gay or a woman affects every aspect of a person's life: if everyone is treated in the same way you can be sure that it is a white, heterosexual male-defined way.

Problems and their solutions can only be understood within the cultural context in which they occur, and the particular stresses, strains, disadvantages, advantages and opportunities that this context affords. It is not possible to understand the experiences of a black Briton outside the context of overt and covert racism and the beliefs, values and attitudes of the black communities which they inhabit. Similarly the life experiences of a lesbian, a gay man, or a woman cannot be understood outside of the context and implications of sexism and heterosexism – being jeered at, beaten up, sacked, disowned by family and friends, rendered invisible – and the resources available within lesbian, gay and women's communities.

If lesbians, and to a lesser extent, gay men, are often oppressed as a consequence of assumptions of heterosexuality that render them, and their lives, invisible, black Britons are often oppressed because of their very visibility. In relation to race, there is a wealth of evidence that mental health services differentially disadvantage black people (Francis et al., 1989). For example, African Caribbeans are more likely to be diagnosed as suffering from schizophrenia (Harrison et al., 1988; King et al., 1994; Perkins and Fisher, 1995a), more likely to be considered dangerous, more likely to be compulsorily detained (Ineichen et al., 1984) in secure settings (DOH, 1993b), and there is a relative under-diagnosis of affective disorders (Harrison et al., 1988). More importantly, Fernando (1991, 1995) refers to the 'categorical fallacy' which is:

> The imposition of one culture's diagnostic categories of illness to patients of another culture.
>
> *Fernando, 1995*

However, the problem is not merely one of categorization, but of the whole construction and manifestation of distress. Different cultures have different expressions of distress that can readily be misunderstood and misconstrued as madness when viewed through another culture's eyes: normal behaviour within one culture can look like mad behaviour within another. Nowhere is this cultural imperialism more evident than in the widespread use of the concept of 'insight' within psychiatry (Perkins and Moodley, 1993b). A person is deemed to have insight if their understanding of their problems and situation is the same as that of their doctor. Aubrey Lewis (1934) defined insight as 'A correct attitude to morbid change in oneself', and David (1990) merely extended this definition to involve not only agreeing with the doctor that one is in fact mentally ill, but also agreeing with the remediation for that illness and reconstructing one's experience within the concepts of western psychiatry.

Within such a eurocentric view of the world, different conceptualizations of distress – in terms, for example, of one's karma or bodily imbalance or disharmony (Eisenbruch, 1990; Blumhagen, 1981; Weiss et al., 1986) – indicate lack of insight. And when a person is deemed to lack insight this gives the mental health worker a justification to disregard what they are saying (because they do not understand what is 'really' going on) and, if necessary, to treat them against their will. The UK encompasses a wide variety of different cultures, beliefs and values, and distress and disturbance can only be understood within the cultural context in which they occur. For a culture whose values and beliefs are at odds with prevailing white norms, the appropriate context is not that afforded by the narrow perspective of scientific psychiatry: the approach most prevalent in UK services but alien to many of the other cultural groups who inhabit these shores.

When the behaviour and experience of oppressed groups is considered mad by a society defined by white, male, heterosexuals, an understandable response of oppressed groups has been, in various ways, to argue 'We're not mad, we're angry': to dissociate themselves from any notion of madness so as not to make more problematic their already difficult and tenuous position. But what does this mean for those lesbians, gay men, women, and blacks who are mad – who are disturbed and distressed by cognitive and emotional problems?

It is undoubtedly the case that some people from oppressed groups are labelled 'mad' inappropriately, for others the stresses and strains of oppression undoubtedly exacerbate cognitive and emotional difficulties, and social disadvantages contribute to disability. In the context of oppression it is not possible to know how much serious social disability there would be in the absence of oppression. However, it is difficult to understand why the processes of thinking and feeling should be any more immune from disability than are other human systems – sight, hearing, mobility and the like. It is undoubtedly the case that oppression exacerbates disability (see Chesler, 1972; Kitzinger and Perkins, 1993; King et al., 1994; Perkins and Fisher, 1995a), but it is often also the sad reality that socially disabled blacks, lesbians, women and gays are doubly excluded. Excluded from black, lesbian, women's and gay male cultures because of their failure to behave in ways considered appropriate in these communities, and from the ascendant white, heterosexual, male culture both because of this social disability and because of their race, culture, gender, lesbianism or homosexuality. Not an enviable position. After returning from a visit to her family, one black lesbian with serious mental health problems said to us:

> Everywhere I'm too far the other side of the tracks – I got to be normal.

Black communities are no more immune from sexism and heterosexism than lesbian communities are immune from racism and gay communities from sexism and racism. This black lesbian therefore had to contend with the racism of lesbian communities and the heterosexism and sexism of black communities ... as well as the racism, sexism and heterosexism of mental health services.

In these services the white, male, heterosexual values of the predominant culture prevail, yet these are the services that confront blacks, women, lesbians and gay men who are seriously socially disabled by ongoing mental health problems. These oppressed peoples adopt different ways of coping and of surviving.

Some reject the norms, values and prescriptions with which they are presented and continue to fight against a system that has labelled them as mad (Perkins and Moodley, 1993a). There then often ensues an intermittent and acrimonious relationship with services that can be extremely destructive for the person concerned. The consequence of rejecting a service often results in their being deemed unmotivated, uncooperative and being rejected by those services. For someone with serious problems this can result in a cycle of compulsory detention, forced treatment and exclusion. The person is hospitalized and medicated against their will when their behaviour cannot be tolerated outside hospital. They leave hospital as soon as they can, some attempt to use ongoing services in a manner that suits them, but this is too often deemed inappropriate and they are banned because of their failure to obey the rules. Others simply reject support in the community from a system that they view as entirely aversive and punitive and are therefore discharged despite their support needs. In either case, they fail to get the support they need, and there is nothing to stop deterioration and further compulsory detention. During this process the person is often excluded from numerous roles and services: work, family, friends, as well as hostels, community centres and drop-ins, who are ill equipped to provide the help and support that is lacking from statutory mental health services. For example: one young black man had been repeatedly admitted to hospital when his family and neighbours could not tolerate his behaviour: he would become very distressed, aggressive to his parents, disruptive to neighbours and steal things from them. During periods of compulsory detention he was treated with drugs and his distress and disturbance did subside, but he loathed the system and would discharge himself as soon as legally possible. At the same time, he had been banned from many mental health service facilities (inside the hospital and outside) because he was disruptive and got into arguments and fights. His relationship with services was one in which staff disliked him because he was seen as 'abusing' the care they tried to offer. He was in the paradoxical position of alternately (and often simultaneously) being banned and compulsorily detained: an incredible situation that he experienced as both punishing and rejecting and not at all supportive or helpful. This man is far from being alone in these experiences and the disastrous cycle set up can all too often lead to suicide or the criminal justice system.

Other people from oppressed groups attempt to comply with the demands of psychiatric services and adopt the norms and expectations of white society. It is not uncommon to find black people claiming that they are white, lesbians and gay men claiming to be heterosexual, just trying to fit in. One young black man with whom we worked went as far as painting his face and body with white paint in his efforts to be white. Many others deny their race and cultural origins in less literal ways, believing, from the evidence of the services with which they are presented, that to be normal and to succeed it is essential to be white. To watch black clients refuse to talk to black staff or call black mental health workers 'black bastard' or 'nigger bitch' is a shocking reflection of the services in which we work.

Similarly, many women adopt the male prescriptions of what they should do. Seriously socially disabled women have often manifestly failed to live up to these expectations – hence their need for long term care from services. This is probably most graphically illustrated in pregnancy and motherhood. In a society which gives pride of place to the institution of motherhood, many disabled women who have not had children feel that they have failed because of this. Younger women may see their only hope of acceptance in lying in becoming a mother, but this can lead to an awful chain of events (Perkins, 1992b). The implicit assumption that 'the mad should not breed' is still widespread, and in the early stages of a pregnancy many women are put under considerable pressure to have an abortion. However, if they resist these exhortations, there follow nine months when they are accorded a status that they have not hitherto enjoyed. They are treated with respect, as a worthwhile person: a mother-to-be. But this role and status are often short lived. For a woman who herself requires a great deal of help and support, there is no provision to offer her a high level of ongoing help to look after her baby as well. We have seen no socially disabled mothers actively harm their babies but we have seen many who are not able to look after them, with the inevitable consequence that the child is taken into care. The child's needs are generally considered to be paramount and often the woman has few real allies in the traumatic process of fostering and adoption that follows. Whilst the child is fostered the mother may be able to retain contact, but it is rare indeed for an open adoption to be arranged which will allow continuing access. Is there any evidence that infrequent supervised visits with a birth mother who has mental health problems are damaging to a child?

The disabled mother not only has to cope with the guilt and failure of losing her child, but her 'failure' as a mother is often greeted with criticism and rejection by family, friends and some mental health workers. To have a child and fail to care for it is often viewed as worse than not having it. In response to these stressors, many women relapse and become acutely distressed and disturbed for protracted periods. Yet others give up and we have known several socially disabled women to have become seriously depressed, even attempting to kill themselves when their child has been taken into care. In addition, or alternatively, we have known numerous disabled women who go on to have other children and get into a tragic cycle: pregnancy affords an attractive and valued role and status for a time – a purpose in life – that is followed by grief and anguish at fostering and adoption. We know one woman who repeated this cycle seven times.

CHALLENGES TO COMMUNITY CARE SERVICES

If services are to begin to accommodate the needs of doubly disadvantaged groups, it goes without saying that everyone must recognize and challenge the white, heterosexual male assumptions that they are making. This cannot be a passive process of acceptance but must be an active process of reconstruction and welcome. To take the view that 'We don't discriminate against anyone here' guarantees that a white, heterosexual, male environment will be maintained.

Ensuring access means different things for different oppressed groups and it is not possible to cover the full range here. However, in general there are two areas that must be considered. First, there is the acceptability of the service settings and facilities, the behaviour of staff within them and liaison with the relevant communities outside mental health services. Making our mental health facilities acceptable means actively showing lesbians, gay men, women, blacks, that they are welcome. This might include the following.

- Putting up posters of lesbians and gay men on the wall, and of key figures and events in the black community.
- Displaying the number of gay switchboard/lesbian line and black organizations and activities.
- Routinely handing out up-to-date leaflets about 'women-only' events and facilities within black and gay communities.
- Setting up groups and activities specifically for lesbians, gays or blacks.
- Offering women-only facilities and activities, trips to black clubs, gay or lesbian bars.
- Inviting local black, gay, lesbian and women's organizations to run activities.
- Celebrating all the major festivals of relevance to the local community, not just the Christian ones.
- Changing initial interviews with a person to ask about all important relationships and actively say 'he or she' to people of both genders.
- Exploring the person's experience of racism, sexism, anti-lesbianism, anti-gay abuse/violence, domestic violence, sexual harassment and assault: all the problems that people from oppressed groups experience, but about which those who are not so oppressed rarely enquire.

The list is almost endless. However, we have often been told that racism and heterosexism are 'not issues in our service'. The argument runs 'We have very few black users' or 'We don't have any lesbian or gay users'. This is fallacious for three reasons. First, in relation to race, it is even more important to make the service acceptable to black users if there are only one or two of them: they are even more isolated and marginalized than if they are in a service with many black users. Second, in relation to lesbians and gays, given psychiatry's heritage of regarding lesbians and gays as pathological *per se*, most users (and most staff) will not 'come out' unless they feel safe to do so: unless they can see that they are in a lesbian/gay-friendly environment. Third, it is likely that some women blacks, lesbians and gays will have been put off using the service because it is so orientated to white, male heterosexuals. We knew of a day centre in a largely African Caribbean area of London where all the attenders were white – and, understandably, any black client referred did not stay long. A lesbian client who once attended a day centre told us:

At the day centre they were always trying to pair me up with men. I'm not interested in men, you know. I like women, but at [the day centre] it's always about men. I left.

Perkins, 1995

Many sheltered/supported work projects are so male dominated that they are not a pleasant place for women with serious mental health problems to work (Perkins and Rowland, 1990). In short, specific attention has to be paid to the needs of women, lesbians, gays, blacks to attract them back to the services they may need and from which they have, by default, been excluded.

Next there is a more detailed understanding of the ways in which distress is manifested and construed in different cultures. In order to understand what help the person needs we need to understand the cultural context in which their problems occur and the solutions that will be acceptable within this context. Sometimes it may be possible to combine western psychiatric interventions with those based on other spiritual or religious paradigms (Perkins and Moodley, 1993a). For example, a young African Caribbean man with whom we worked was extremely distressed because he was unable to pray. His problems, within western psychiatry, were understood as the disturbances of thought characteristic of schizophrenia. This young man both believed in both physical and spiritual models of his problems, and a combination of neuroleptics (to help him to think more clearly so he could pray) and attendance at healing services at a Pentecostal church (which did much to reduce his anxiety and guilt at having problems praying) went a long way to alleviating his distress and helping him cope with his difficulties.

Whilst a great deal has been written about the misuse of drugs, it is important to remember that talking therapies are no less eurocentric: no less based on white, male, heterosexual beliefs about human experience. Psychotherapies based on heterosexual assumptions, like analytic models, are oppressive to lesbians and gay men. Models based on the desirability of western concepts like free will and choice are incompatible with cultures where obligation and determinism are more important values. Most psychotherapies are predicated on the assumption that it is a good thing to express one's feelings: inappropriate for people from cultures where this is considered a very undesirable thing to do.

It is also important to recognize those things that are important to people of different groups and cultures. For example, the acceptance and encouragement of a lesbian partner, the recognition of relationships. The importance of relationships other than that with her husband to a disturbed woman: many heterosexual women have very close and important female friends. The head covering of a Moslem woman and the bathing, showering and hygiene preferences of those from different cultures. The dates and requirements of different festivals and religious obligations are also central.

At times of acute disturbance and distress a person may not be able to articulate their beliefs and needs, therefore it can be helpful to have links with others important to the person and their local community and gain the necessary information. However, it is important, in this context, to remember that we do not all do what our priest, our parents or others who are significant in our lives believe that we should. We have, for example, found many Jamaican parents who are appalled by their British born sons' Rastafarianism.

Most of all, in creating 'community-based' services, we need to become more sophisticated in thinking about what 'community' means. Within mental health services, 'community' is typically taken to mean anywhere outside the hospital. 'The community' is not, however, a physical location. Sometimes, community is defined by its geography, as in 'the group of people who live in this street', but more often it is defined by a set of common interests, character-istics, roles and circumstances. Communities are defined by the relationships of their members so that most people are part of several communities: a commu-nity of colleagues at work, mothers at the playgroup, drinkers at the pub, Labour Party members, a tenant's association: groups of more or less like-minded people with whom we identify ourselves, with whom we share experi-ences and who identify us as being part of the group. Some of these identities are more important than others.

Moving away from the concept of community as 'anywhere outside hospi-tal', it is important to start looking at the relevant communities for all clients. This is particularly critical for those clients from oppressed groups because the default option, when the community is treated as anywhere outside hospital, is white, heterosexual and male. It is necessary that we explore how black, lesbian, gay and women's communities can be made accessible for our clients. But simplistic notions must be avoided. Too often it is assumed that there is 'a' lesbian or 'a' black community. This is not true. There are numerous different lesbian, gay, black and women's communities, and whilst there may be some overlap, each has different beliefs, politics, values and organizations.

Texts about community care stress the importance of understanding the resources available in 'the community' (Rapp and Wintersteen, 1989). Actually, we need to know about the resources available in a range of different communi-ties, to explore clients' values and beliefs and ensure that they can gain access to those communities and facilities that are relevant to them. Sometimes, if a person has been out of circulation for some time, they may want or need to explore a range of different communities.

Finally, if communities are groups of people who identify themselves in particular ways and who share important beliefs, characteristics, values and experiences, then an important community for people with serious mental health problems may be others who have similar difficulties. Much of normalization theory devalues these relationships by suggesting that people should share places and have relationships with 'valued citizens': those who do not have mental health problems (Wolfensberger and Tullman, 1982). This approach is devaluing of those who have experienced mental health problems. Many people with such difficulties are becoming part of the growing user/survivor move-ments – and have valued and valuable roles in important arenas. For those users who are from other oppressed groups, networks of, for example, black users and lesbian survivors are developing. These communities of users, independent and apart from mental health professionals and the services they inhabit, have a vital role to play on the mental health scene.

The disenfranchised and the disliked: those whom services fail

14

Mental health services currently fail people from oppressed groups but, over the past decade, great concern has also been expressed about those who 'fall through the net' of community services (see Bachrach, 1982; Showalter, 1987; Ritchie *et al.*, 1994; Repper and Perkins, 1995). Studies have shown that some 40–50% of people with serious long term mental health problems either reject or drop-out of services or 'underutilize' them by taking up only some of the support offered (Bender and Pilling, 1985; Meltzer *et al.*, 1991). However, the expression 'fall through the net' can be misleading.

Some people simply never come into contact with services. Others do not avail themselves of services they are offered because their disabilities prevent them from doing so. There is little point in sending someone an appointment letter if they are unable to read or expect them to arrive for an out-patient appointment if their level of cognitive disorganization or lack of money for the fare makes it difficult, if not impossible, for them to do so. Yet others, often those who have had past experience of compulsory treatment, actively avoid and reject support and services because they find them unacceptable. Finally, there are a number of people who are actively excluded from services because mental health workers consider them to be unsuitable or to have abused that which is offered (Bachrach, 1982; Repper and Perkins, 1995). People who make constant demands on services, who use many different services at the same time (often telling each that they have no other form of help) and who become angry and abusive when they do not receive the support they want, are often banned from services. This can leave them barely able to survive in the community, or cause them to enter penal or homeless facilities which are ill equipped to meet their needs. There are many services that have an informal, or a formal, 'black-list' (*sic*) of people whom they will under no circumstances allow through their doors (Bachrach, 1989). We have experienced situations where this list is held by the duty senior nurse and any proposed admissions checked against it in the manner of stolen credit cards.

Whilst it is probably the case that some of those people who are rejected by, or who fail to take up, long term care services do so because they do not need support, for the majority this does not appear to be the case. Studies have shown that many of these people end up:

- Living in impoverished conditions (Johnstone *et al.*, 1984);
- Socially isolated (Beels *et al.*, 1984);
- With untreated physical health problems (Koran *et al.*, 1989; Wells *et al.*, 1989);
- Homeless (Timms and Fry, 1989; Weller, 1989);
- At risk of physical violence and exploitation (Bachrach, 1985);
- Falling foul of the criminal justice system (Coid, 1988; Maden *et al.*, 1994);
- Spending a great deal of their time doing absolutely nothing (Warden *et al.*, 1990); and
- Posing great risk to themselves through self-harm and suicide and to others. This has resulted in several enquiries, such as that into the murder of Mr Zito by Christopher Clunis (Ritchie *et al.*, 1994): a man whom psychiatric services had manifestly failed over a protracted period of time.

Such people find services unacceptable and services find them unacceptable. They are often actively disliked by mental health workers because they fail to take the advice they give, are often aggressive and rude, sometimes demanding, and frequently engage in behaviour that service providers consider self-destructive. Often these clients are deemed by mental health workers to be undeserving of help (Repper and Perkins, 1995). Hirsch (1992, p. 4) have described them as:

> A group of patients who are hard to sustain in a meaningful clinical alliance with psychiatric services ... These patients do not engage in treatment, are often not at home when the doctors, nurses or social workers visit, and may abuse alcohol [or drugs] ... They sometimes end up with no home of their own.

A DIAGNOSTIC CHALLENGE

One of the most important features of people who are rejected by, or who reject, services is the nature of their difficulties. Many have a controversial diagnosis of some form of 'personality disorder' in addition to, or instead of, their mental health problems: a diagnosis that reflects both problems in coping with everyday life and relationships and a failure to use support services, or a style of service use that is deemed by service providers as abuse. For example, one young man had ongoing cognitive and emotional problems, rarely talked to staff except to tell them to 'fuck off', drank as much alcohol as his limited income would allow (and stole money to get more when this ran out) and was frequently violent to other service users or staff whom he thought had interfered with him. However, even a cursory look at his past revealed that he had an appalling childhood: found at the age of five starving in a flat with his brothers and no sign then or since of parents, shuffled between some 10 foster homes between this time and the end of his childhood years, during the course of which he was excluded from school and received very little education. In diagnostic terms he was considered to have a 'personality disorder', but this might best be understood in terms of his childhood having left him with few personal or material resources and having no reason to trust anyone. His experience of services had been little different: he had been rejected by a variety of different facilities and almost universally engendered dislike in those who worked with him.

A similar lack of personal, social and material resources could be seen in a young woman who had been dumped on the motorway at the age of seven, grew up in care and, between the ages of 18 and 24, had been thrown out of four social services hostels, two voluntary sector hostels and two sets of bed and breakfast accommodation, interspersed with admissions to psychiatric hospital. This woman had received a variety of diagnoses. Initially considered to have a major affective disorder, her 'manipulative' behaviour (often causing havoc in the staff group by setting staff against each other) and self-harm (invariably met with staff ignoring her with the idea that if they attended to her wounds they would be reinforcing her behaviour) had eventually caused this to be reformulated as 'personality disorder'. This diagnostic reformulation had on several occasions led to her discharge (a point to which we will return later). She found it almost impossible to trust people: her history both within and outside mental health services had provided her with numerous lessons that people always let you down. She was completely alone in the world except for a series of transient boyfriends from whom she gained, in physical terms, the emotional warmth and security she had always lacked.

There are numerous more examples we could give of people with lives and problems like these; some remain compulsorily detained in hospitals, others continue to seek help but do so in ways that services do not like. Some use multiple different services. One of the key issues that mental health services have to address is 'Who are we designed to serve?' There is rarely any question that people who have received a diagnosis of schizophrenia or bipolar affective disorder should have service input. The problems tend to arise when these diagnoses are replaced with, or co-occur with, diagnoses of 'personality disorder'. There are many continuing community care services that erect barriers such as 'We do not take people with personality disorders'. Alternatively, conditions are set on the use of services that amount to the restriction that 'We only take people who will abide by the rules' (not being disruptive, not using drugs/alcohol, attending meetings, groups and activities, etc.) that many such people cannot, or do not want to, meet.

Taking a slightly cynical perspective, it often seems that the necessary 'meal ticket' diagnoses for receipt of continuing community care are those of psychotic or major affective illness and the 'sacking' diagnoses are those of 'alcohol or drug misuse', 'drug-induced psychosis' and 'personality disorder'. In relation to 'personality disorder', mental health services tend to have a double standard. Whilst a person can be detained in a psychiatric hospital against their will (a diagnosis of personality disorder is included in mental health legislation as a reason for compulsory admission and treatment), they can also be excluded from community care services because they are deemed not to be mentally ill but to have a 'personality disorder'.

This diagnostic catch-22 is probably maintained because of the understandable wish to exclude those people who are disturbing, disruptive and difficult to help. It is not easy to provide services for people who are often rootless, frequently claim that there is nothing wrong with them (despite making what are considered excessive demands on services), lack any desire to change and present challenging behaviours that render them unacceptable to other service users (Hirsch, 1992). However, this situation also reflects a tension between illness and social models. If one adopts a strict illness model of mental health problems then there is no question that people with 'personality problems' would be excluded. However, it is clear in mental health legislation that society wishes to maintain the right to compulsorily detain people who behave in unacceptable ways but who did not fit into the mental illness categories available.

Throughout this text we have emphasized that a social disability model is necessary for understanding and helping people who have ongoing mental health problems. A person requires ongoing support, not because of their cognitive and emotional difficulties *per se*, but because of the effect of these, together with the stigma and rejection they experience, on their role functioning. Mental health problems are a socially-defined phenomenon: people are deemed by others, or deem themselves, to need help when they are not able to cope and behave in ways that are acceptable within the society in which they live.

There is not infrequently a conflict between what society and mental health professionals consider to constitute madness. Society can deem someone to be mad when mental health workers do not: a situation which often occurs in relation to those deemed to have 'personality disorder'. For example, despite an initial diagnosis of bipolar affective illness, a young woman was reassessed and considered to have a personality disorder. She was discharged against her will and the discharge we witnessed was quite spectacular. She was escorted to the gate by two security guards wearing only a black lace bra and knickers, followed by a nurse carrying her clothes and other belongings to the gate. There then followed a somewhat bizarre series of events: a tussle between the local community and mental health services. She lay down on the railway tracks, the police were called and she was taken to hospital where she was deemed not to be mentally ill and sent away. She lay down on the road, distraught drivers called the police and the same sequence of events was repeated. She threw all the furniture out of her second floor flat. Worried neighbours called the police and the cycle was repeated again. Clearly, the community in which she lived deemed her to be mad because of her behaviour but the diagnostic systems employed by psychiatry disagreed with this. This saga ended in a somewhat ironical fashion which illustrates the contradictions involved. When refused admission on the third occasion of assessment she attacked the doctor. As a consequence of this she was compulsorily admitted. She did not want to leave hospital in the first place, she did her best to get back in and she ended up being compulsorily detained.

If mental health problems are considered within a social disability framework then such diagnostic exclusions would not arise. A person needs help from services if they are unable to live up to the standards they expect of themselves and that others expect of them (Wing and Morris, 1981), irrespective of their diagnosis. Such people are not well served within the homelessness or crimi-nolegal networks, but they can be supported within community mental health services if these services are prepared to take them and adapt to their needs.

In our opinion, it is probably most helpful to consider those personality disorders that render a person unable to cope with everyday life and relationships as reflecting a lack of the personal (and often social and material) resources that are necessary for effective role functioning. People who lack these resources have specific difficulties in forming and maintaining relationships and activities. They may not benefit from medication, but there are many other social and psychological supports and interventions which can help. Clearly, if someone has this type of difficulty in addition to other mental health problems (as have many recipients of long term community care services) then this lack of personal resources makes it very much more difficult for them to cope with their cognitive and emotional difficulties and social disadvantages.

THE CHALLENGER AND THE CHALLENGED: A STRUGGLE FOR POWER

Issues of power are probably at the heart of mental health service's failure to meet the needs of those considered to have 'personality disorders'. In former times staff were very clearly in control within institutions which were often run for the convenience of these staff rather than for their therapeutic value. In community-focused services staff retain a great deal of power and many are reluctant to give it up, which means that problems arise when service users either refuse to accept that power or challenge it. We described earlier the case of a woman who did not want to be discharged from hospital, who did her best to get back in and was eventually compulsorily admitted. The chain of events described could be seen as illustrating a power struggle. She said she wanted to stay in hospital and did her best to do so, to the point of refusing to get dressed. Staff believed that they knew best: they had decided that she did not have a bipolar affective disorder but a personality disorder for which hospitalization was inappropriate: they therefore discharged her. She tried to get back, but the staff saw her as being 'manipulative' (lying on the railway line/road and throwing her furniture out of her window) and therefore would not admit her. However, when she became violent whilst being assessed they could once again exercise control by compulsorily admitting her.

Mental health workers do not like to feel that they are being controlled by service users – often using the terms 'manipulative behaviour' or 'attention seeking' when they feel that this is happening. It is important to emphasize several factors about the control that mental health professionals exercise.

First, power is not solely rested in the hands of senior clinicians or within one professional group. It is easy for other mental health workers to say 'The doctors have all the power', or for junior staff to say 'The senior staff have all the power' or for clinical staff to say 'The managers have all the power'. In no case is this correct. Staff may feel powerless, but all are more powerful within mental health services than the clients whom they serve.

Second, this control does not emanate exclusively from mental health legislation. Compulsory detention and treatment are only a small part of the control that mental health workers exert, but constitute an important back up threat (explicit or implicit) to increase the effectiveness of other forms of power: 'If you don't do this then we might have to section you'. The ways in which professionals exercise power are many and various and often derive from honourable, if misguided, motives.

- **Withdrawal of approval.** Most people want to be liked by those around them and seek to behave in ways that elicit approval. The giving and removal of approval is therefore an important way of exercising control. A mental health worker may therefore exercise their power by withdrawing attention and concern when a person does something of which they disapprove. This can take many forms: ceasing to respond to approaches or requests, not speaking to the person or avoiding them, actively criticizing them or simply becoming more cold and distant. This may be linked with withdrawal of services contingent upon particular behaviours: 'I will only come and visit you if you take your medication', 'You can only live here if you do not drink', 'You can only have lunch here if you join in with one of the groups'.
- **The giving of privileges.** For example, 'If you go to the day centre I will take you out to the pub tonight' is a strategy often graced with the term 'behavioural programme', but is both ethically dubious and clinically disadvantageous. A person's rights are infringed if the only way they can do something they want to do is by also doing something that they do not want. There is also the risk that the person will fail to do two things that the mental health worker considers desirable rather than one: not go to the day centre or

the pub. In general, one desirable behaviour should never be made contingent on another.

- **Verbal persuasion** is another particularly potent form of power, especially when a client is less well informed and less articulate than the mental health worker. Mental health professionals have access to a great deal of information but it is very common for them only to impart a small proportion of this to clients in an attempt to sway their decisions in the direction that the clinician has decided.

- **Contracts** are a popular way of withdrawing support if people do not use services as they are intended. Such contracts specify the conditions on which a person can use a service and are typically written down and signed by staff and client in a quasi-legal agreement. They might say, for example, you can only go to the workshop if you arrive at 9.00 am every morning, do not come in drunk and do not upset other workers. The sanction for breaking these conditions is almost invariably withdrawal of the service: being sacked from the workshop. It is our view that such contracts are not helpful to the individual concerned. They represent a way of getting rid of those whom mental health workers cannot control as well as depriving these people of the support they need unless they accept the service on terms defined by staff. For example, one man referred to us had a contract on the acute ward where he was a patient. It said that he could only stay there if he went to the sheltered workshop every day. He signed this agreement and then broke it two weeks later. He was duly discharged (as per the contract) and returned to hospital by the police four days later having been found wandering naked in the street.

Power struggles are often at the root of the problems that services have in providing effective support for those groups whom they currently fail. Many people with serious ongoing mental health problems accept mental health workers' power and prescriptions, but this is not necessarily a good thing. Such acceptance can be at high cost in terms of the individual's self-confidence and trust in their own judgements. Indeed, we have seen many people 'institutionalized' by community care services in much the same manner as they were in the old institutions: one man in his middle years recently asked our permission to invite a friend round to his flat – his own flat – for tea.

Those who abuse or reject services, or fail to do what mental health workers say, typically enter a power struggle to get the support they want on their own terms, or to avoid any kind of association with services. However, there are many ways in which these people represent a success of community care services, although they are rarely perceived in this way. Despite their problems and support needs many retain a pride, independence, confidence in their judgements and ordinary expectations that in someone who does not have mental health problems would be wholly desirable. Unless services can enable people

to receive support whilst retaining these desirable qualities, community care
will have failed.

THE SHORTCOMINGS OF COMPULSION

A common response to those seriously socially disabled people who abuse or
fail to use services is to call for greater powers of compulsion: more power to
insist that people do things that mental health workers think are good for them.
There has been much popular and political concern over people who will not
use services, who end up in prisons or homeless, especially the very small
number who commit violent crimes. In this context it is worth pointing out that
people with serious ongoing mental health problems are more likely to be
victims of violent crimes than they are to commit them. In the long term care
service in which one of us works, 80% of users had been victims of physical
assault (Perkins and Prince, 1993). However, neglect and violence are of
concern and the issue is whether more compulsion provides an answer.

Mental health services have always had the power to compulsorily treat
people. However, in the UK this has hitherto been restricted to treatment in
psychiatric hospitals. Community care has meant that most people who experience serious mental health problems are no longer resident in hospitals and
when they are not in hospitals they cannot be compulsorily treated. There has
been a change in support settings but no parallel change in legal powers to
control. This imbalance has led many to calls for increased powers to compel
people to accept treatment and support in the community: such powers already
exist in some areas of the USA and have been considered in the UK (DOH,
1993b). The essence of these developments is a desire to further extend the
power of mental health professionals outside a hospital setting.

We would argue that these moves are problematic. If a person does not want
to accept help and support outside hospital, or does not want to accept it in the
manner designed, then they are unlikely to be persuaded that the help is a good
idea by being forced to accept it. If a person is living in their own flat and
mental health staff have a right to enter that flat and, for example, compulsorily
medicate them, the possibility of developing a trusting relationship is diminished. It is likely that the person will endeavour to be out when the professional
calls and may avoid contact by moving out completely, rendering themselves
homeless and completely without support. Increased compulsion is likely to
decrease acceptance of support and worsen the person's relationship with
mental health services, aggravating a vicious cycle that already exists in
'revolving door' compulsory hospitalization. The more you force someone to do
something, the less they will trust you and the less they will be prepared to
accept your support.

Compulsion could also be seen as offering a licence for poor practice. It takes
time and effort to form good working relationships with people, especially those

who services find challenging. Compulsion may offer an attractive short cut that obviates the need for such effort. But it is a short-sighted strategy making future relationship formation and support even more difficult. Further, compulsion in the community could be seen as racist because it is likely to be differentially applied to different groups – especially African Caribbeans. We know that mental health services already have a poor relationship with African Caribbean communities (Confederation of Indian Organisations, 1992; Lowe, 1992; MIND, 1994) and that a much higher proportion of African Caribbean users are compulsorily detained under existing legislation (see Moodley and Perkins, 1991). Extrapolating from the present situation, if compulsion were extended to a community setting it is likely that a higher proportion of African Caribbeans would be subject to its prescriptions. An already poor relationship would be further worsened and the service received by African Caribbeans would markedly deteriorate.

Most citizens have the right to accept or refuse health care. If we are prescribed a drug or an operation that we think is not going to be in our interests we refuse it, but people who are considered to have mental health problems are not accorded these rights. It is generally assumed that a person deemed mentally ill is unable to make rational decisions and requires someone else to take decisions for them. This extends to providing them with treatment, against their will if necessary.

There will be occasions when a person's behaviour cannot be tolerated and difficult legal and ethical decisions must be made that involve balancing the role of providing treatment and support for the individual, and that of social control and protection of the public. This is made all the more complex by the divergent views of different interest groups. Frequently attempts are made to gain the agreement of all involved: users, providers, relatives, general practitioners, local community organizations and so forth. Although it is clear that all of these groups have a stake in mental health services, it is often not possible to reach consensus decisions (Shepherd et al., 1994). There is a tension between, for example, users (who want their rights respected and support on their own terms), relatives (who want respite from the 'burden' of providing care and a 'safe place' for their kin), a local community (who want to witness minimal disruption in their area and a knowledge that those who are disturbed are being cared for) and the police (who want someone to take difficult people off their hands as quickly as possible).

Differences must be recognized and debated: efforts to achieve a cosy consensus simply obscure the diversity of interests. It is also important to recognize that these considerations are not primarily mental health issues, rather they are moral, ethical and social debates. This distinction is important. Any citizen can have a view and to some extent contribute (through various electoral, lobbying and legal channels) to debates and decisions about what is right and wrong. However, if a decision becomes a medical or a psychiatric one then it becomes the province of medical and psychiatric experts only. We are not convinced that doctors should be in a position to make moral judgements on behalf of the rest of society in the guise of psychiatric expertise. Psychiatrists, despite their many skills, are not experts in ethics, nor are there political constraints upon their judgements.

The issue of whether people with mental health problems should be sent to prison if they have committed a crime falls into this category of complex socio–ethical, medico–legal dilemmas. Clearly there are concerns about people being inappropriately incarcerated in jails, but there are also concerns about the treatment they receive in special high-security psychiatric institutions. It is worth noting that many service users are of the opinion they would rather go to prison than be compulsorily detained in hospital. We have been told that you get treated better in prison, that it is less stigmatizing to go to prison than psychiatric hospital and that at least a prison sentence has a time limit whereas detention under a court section of mental health legislation does not. Clearly, the balance between criminal responsibility and mental health problems is a fine one, but we would argue that there is a case for further separation of legal detention for a crime and for mental health problems. If someone with cognitive and emotional problems commits a crime then it is up to the courts whether they should be locked up. If the decision is made that custody is necessary then responsibility for this should rest with the penal system leaving mental health treatment and support the province of mental health services. It is not possible to see penal facilities as simply another 'community' in which mental health care and support can be provided.

If people are diverted from penal services to mental health services when they commit crimes this has several negative effects. First, mental health services have the dual role of acting as jailer and therapist: it is difficult to act in the client's interests when one also has a legal obligation to act in the interest of the public and keep them safe. The psychiatric hospital becomes a prison. Second, it maintains the popular belief that people with mental health problems are all dangerous and thus disadvantages others who experience these difficulties. Most people who have serious ongoing mental health problems do not commit crimes and are not dangerous. Whilst a person's mental health problems may have contributed to their crimes, it is very rare indeed that these problems can be seen as the sole cause. Third, it can be demeaning to people with serious mental health problems to deny that they have any agency or control over their actions.

Many people with serious mental health problems who come to the attention of courts fall into the group who we reject, or are considered to abuse the supports and treatment available. A study of enquiries into legal cases concerning people with mental health problems (Zito Trust, 1995) clearly suggests that if more acceptable and effective outreach services were provided then much violent and offending behaviour could be prevented.

FACING THE CHALLENGE: MEETING PEOPLE ON THEIR OWN TERMS

Many people have written about improving services for those who exhibit challenging behaviour and turn down the support they need (Bachrach, 1982; Hirsch, 1992; Repper and Perkins, 1995). Relationships are probably the key issue. Most people who are reluctant to engage in mental health care have every reason to be suspicious of services. This may arise because they have never been able to trust anyone in their lives, or because their experience of mental health services has been one of compulsion and forced treatment: hardly the best basis of a productive relationship. Alternatively, they may have been rejected by services when they felt they needed them. Rarely have they experienced in mental health services someone who is on their side, someone who likes and values them, stands up for them when others are being critical, someone who will be there no matter where they are or what they do. Often they have been passed from one service to another, from one agency to another: it is someone with a commitment and persistence to stick with them that is important.

But forming such relationships is not easy. Many of the issues that we have already discussed in Part Two are of relevance. In addition to genuinely being able to see value and worth in the client, it is important that mental health workers try to take the person's views seriously and act upon them. Many have had their opinions ignored or misconstrued for many years: forming a good relationship means reversing this. There is no hope of a person learning to trust a relationship if that relationship is unreliable. This includes actually being there when you say you will be there, apologizing personally and in advance if you have to cancel and having a very long time scale. It can take years to undo the damage to a person's ability to form relationships that has been wrought within and outside mental health services. It is easy to feel that one is getting nowhere and give up. However, such giving up would not even leave the person in the same situation as when you started: they would be worse off. Every failed relationship, everyone who lets a person down, makes it harder for them to form relationships in the future. Finally, it is of primary importance to offer the person the help that **they** think they need. It is only by doing this that it is possible to convince them that there is something in mental health services for them.

It is not uncommon for those who challenge services also to manifest 'challenging behaviours'. A common problem is self-destructive behaviour or self-harm. One young woman repeatedly cut herself and the procedure that followed was very predictable: she would be stitched up (often grudgingly) in the Accident and Emergency Department and then be admitted to a psychiatric hospital. There, staff would see her behaviour as 'attention seeking' and therefore would ignore her further threats and attempts to harm herself (except to provide the minimum medical assistance), on the basis that attending to her self-harm would only encourage her. She became frustrated because everyone was ignoring her, she would cut herself more, hit staff and set several fires. Eventually she was discharged because her behaviour could not be contained and before long the cycle repeated itself.

Eventually she was referred to a unit for people with challenging behaviour where a quite different approach was taken: we call it 'non-contingent TLC (tender loving care)'. The main premises of this approach are as follows.

- If a person is harming themself or hitting people, or being disruptive, they are doing so for a reason and that reason is usually acute personal distress. It is important to explore and address the reasons for this.
- If someone is seeking attention then they need attention.
- If someone is seeking attention in ways that we do not like then they have been deprived of more acceptable ways of getting the attention they need.
- It is better to give someone attention as a matter of course than put them in a position where violence and self-harm are the only ways they have to decrease their frustration and express their feelings.

Within non-contingent TLC, staff give a person positive attention (talking to them about their lives, listening to their concerns and problems, doing things they want with them) irrespective of their behaviour. The aim of this is to obviate the need for self-harm/disruptive behaviour. This non-contingent TLC approach has certain advantages. First, it helps the person to see that they are valued: worthy of attention as of right, not dependent on specific things that they do. Everyone needs to feel that someone likes them, is on their side, no matter what, and people with serious mental health problems are no different. Second, non-contingent TLC can serve to resolve some of the problems that lead to the person's self-harm/disruptive behaviour in the first place. By talking to a person about their life, aspiration and problems – understanding why they do the things they do – the underlying cause of their distress can be identified and addressed.

People are not told to refrain from self-harm or disruptive behaviours: these are often functional for the individual concerned. Self-harm is often a way of coping with intolerable distress. Violence and other disruptive behaviours can have a similar effect or be ways of venting frustrations and anxieties that cannot be put into words. Instead of telling a person not to do these things they are asked to try to tell staff – talk to them – before they do them. In the context of receiving non-contingent TLC, many people become able to seek the support of mental health workers as an alternative means of dealing with their problems.

If a person does harm themselves or become disruptive then staff are particularly instructed not to adopt a punitive stance. Instead they explore, in a concerned and non-judgemental manner, how the person felt and why they did what they did. This may seem to be reinforcing undesirable behaviour but this is not a problem because the person receives the same attention and concern at other times so it is not specifically contingent on self-harm/disruptive behaviours.

Further, it is worth pointing out that most people have been 'told off' a great many times (usually under the guise of 'counselling' them) but, since the behaviour is ongoing, this approach has clearly not been effective.

Whether in relation to disruptive behaviours or simply as a way of engaging someone who is reluctant to accept support, the type of non-conditional positive regard and non-conditional attention and concern of this approach are often useful. One young black man was admitted on a section when his behaviour was intolerable outside, received drugs to which he responded, and soon started going round different hospital wards and departments pestering people, stealing things, getting into fights, etc. He would then be discharged and banned from the hospital site but would continue to attend regularly, cause problems and then be evicted. When his mental state worsened he was again compulsorily admitted. Belatedly efforts were made to change this pattern. As he had so often been evicted from mental health services it was made clear that he was more than welcome at the hospital and was helped to make his room homely: within a week it was replete with wall-hangings, posters, bells and cuddly toys. As compulsion had also been a theme in his service history, it was made clear that he could come and go as he pleased, but in order to communicate our concern for his well-being he was asked to either come back at night or let staff know where he was. Compliance with medication had always been an issue and in discussing this it became clear that he was concerned about impotence and hated injections. He asked if he could take pills instead and staff readily acceded to his request: this was the first time he had ever asked for medication. He took the pills religiously. It was not long before he was regularly spending seven nights a week at his girlfriend's house, although he came daily to the hospital, of his own volition, for meals and slept there if he had a row with his girlfriend. A year later this pattern continued, but he had stopped sleeping at the hospital and the time he spent there had decreased. Because he had somewhere in the hospital where he was welcome, and that he could use on his own terms, he was able to live in the community, his disruptive behaviour stopped and he was unbanned from most areas.

This example illustrates several important factors in breaking the destructive vicious cycle of compulsion and rejection.

- Analysing where the relationship between client and mental health services has broken down and taking steps to breach the rift. The focus must be on how services can change to meet the client, not on how the client can change to 'fit in'. In the above example, it was necessary to both make the young man feel welcome and stop dictating what he should and should not do.
- Listening to the client's own concerns and acceding to their requests in order to ensure that they receive the support they want rather than that which others deem necessary. Few of us would continue to use any service that ignored our wishes and failed to provide what we wanted.
- Flexible provision and use of services is the only way in which it is possible

to meet the needs of a diverse group of disabled people, especially those whom services currently fail. Rules and regulations governing the use of community services constitute 'block treatment' which excludes those who do not wish to, or cannot, meet the prescriptions laid down. 'Bending the rules' is required to meet individual needs. The young man described above wanted to maintain contact with the hospital between admissions but day attendance on residential units was not 'allowed'. His attempts to attend the hospital had previously been met with his being banned – and effective support jeopardized for the sake of organizational considerations.

Taking responsibility for failure, acceding to clients' wishes and adapting services to meet their individual needs changes the balance of power between mental health workers and staff. Services need to promote and foster the positive qualities in those whom they currently find challenging: pride, determination, expectations of an ordinary life. If this is to be achieved then compulsion is not the answer: increased force drives disabled people away from the support they need. Mental health workers can and must face the challenge of abandoning attempts to control those whom they cannot and should not control. It is a mistake to assume that mental health services appropriately meet the needs of those who currently use them in the manner determined by professionals. Meeting the challenges posed by those whom current services manifestly fail is important in increasing the accessibility and acceptability of support for all service users.

This type of flexibility in use of services is essential: the more rules and regulations with which we can dispense, the more likely we are to be able to adequately serve those whom we currently fail. However, letting people use services and accept treatments as they want means us giving up power. We need to begin to provide support in our clients' terms and to organize our services around them: allowing people to use services in the ways they want to use them. Clearly, the wants of some service users will be different from those of others, but it is often possible to provide different things for different people in the same setting and eventually to develop new facilities if these are necessary. There are many ways of reducing the 'block treatment' in community services that effectively excludes those who do not wish to, or who cannot, meet the rules and obligations of the setting. Sometimes it may be a question of developing new services, but more often it is a question of using supports flexibly to enable people to avail themselves of the facilities and opportunities that already exist within communities.

There is much of value in the pride and determination of those people whom we currently find challenging. Our challenge is to provide the support that people need to capitalize on these strengths. If this is to be achieved, compulsion is not the answer – it merely worsens relationships and drives people further away. For mental health workers this means facing the challenge of giving up attempting to control those whom we cannot, and should not, control: putting our services at the disposal of those who require support rather than telling them what to do.

Beyond beds: becoming a part of the community | 15

Community care involves not only the discharge of patients from hospitals, but also the discharge of staff and resources, and many of the services that exist have been developed in the context of attempts to close large mental institutions. These institutions provided, albeit in an unsatisfactory manner, a wide range of functions for their inhabitants (Bachrach, 1989): a place to live, work and a variety of leisure pursuits and social opportunities. Whilst accommodation, work, leisure and social relationships are all important for most people, the exigencies of closing a hospital, dictate priority is usually given to the provision of alternative places for people to live. It is important to note that, for most people, a sense of self, identity and esteem is provided less by where they sleep at night than what they do whilst they are awake: their work, relationships and leisure activities.

Resources and support devoted to relationships, work and leisure pursuits may increase the quality of people's lives but they do not close hospitals, or at least their effect on decreasing disability is unlikely to decrease the need for sheltered or supported accommodation on the time scale necessary. As hospital populations decrease, so many of the social, work and leisure activities that they provided cease to function in the face of dwindling numbers. At the same time, the cost per person of continuing hospitalization rises and the need for a speedy closure increases. In 1995 there is something immoral about spending over £100 000 per year to accommodate someone in the back ward of a remote psychiatric institution when the same amount of money would keep four people in a 24-hour staffed domestic house in the community, or provide the much needed intensive outreach support to maintain at least 10 people in their own accommodation.

In the context of closing large hospitals many of the community services thus created continue to revolve around beds: beds in community sheltered and supported accommodation rather than in hospitals. This has two consequences. First, there has been a paucity in the development of work, social and leisure opportunities, and it is not uncommon to find that people have less access to these activities than they had in the large hospitals (Gilman, 1987; Birch, 1983). Second, the focus on provision of sheltered and supported accommodation draws resources away from the support services necessary to prevent people needing to live in special accommodation in the first place. Whilst hostels and supported community houses may represent an improvement on life in a hospital ward, very few of us would choose to live in such group settings. Like anyone else, most people with serious mental health problems want a place of their own: it is towards this end that services must now develop.

THEIR BEDS FOR OURS

The run down of large hospitals and reprovision of supported and sheltered homes outside hospital has led to a shift in resources and a great upheaval for mental health workers and clients alike. Nevertheless, whilst staff and funds are tied up in the supported housing created to replace the hospitals, there are often insufficient resources committed towards preventing people needing supported accommodation and a ludicrous situation develops.

If services for people who experience serious ongoing mental health problems are based on supported accommodation then people will only be referred to such services when they have lost their accommodation. Often they have failed to cope in their own accommodation, but it is also the case that they have rarely received anything like the intensive support necessary to make a success of living in these settings. Having lost their accommodation they move into a supported setting provided by mental health services, where the aim is to help them get back to living in their own place if at all possible. There is something quite criminal about having to wait until someone has lost something before they are helped to get it back, with all the distress, disturbance and sheer waste of time that this process involves. Nevertheless, it is a situation that prevails in an unfortunately high number of services. For example, one man was thrown out of his parental home when he was 19 years old, shortly after his first breakdown when he had became very aggressive towards his father. He was in and out of acute wards for the next 10 years and, in between admissions, he received the standard fortnightly visits from a CPN and quarterly outpatient appointments with the psychiatrist (which he was rarely able to attend). He lived in a variety of different places. Initially he was placed in temporary bed and breakfast accommodation, then in a hostel (from which he was evicted), then back to bed and breakfast before being given his own tenancy. He liked having his own place and managed to stay there for over a year, but the flat became increasingly dirty and sank into a state of disrepair. The neighbours complained that it was an eyesore and lowered the tone of the neighbourhood. He lost weight because he found it difficult to manage his money and buy food and eventually he was evicted, went back to bed and breakfast, then to three different sets of supported lodgings before the last one finally kicked him out. He was not good at communal living and kept getting into arguments and fights with fellow residents. This last eviction left him with nowhere to go but the mental health services. He was referred to a specialist continuing care team who found him a place in a small staffed group home and he began to work towards regaining the home of his own he so desired. It took three years to get back to where he had been 10 years previously: 10 years when his life had been extremely chaotic. He only remains there by virtue of a very high level of support and periodic short readmissions when things get too much for him. He now receives at least thrice weekly visits from a mental health support worker, who helps him to collect his money, buy food, clean his flat, pay bills and all the other requirements of a tenancy. He attends a drop-in for lunch whenever he wants, can (and does) call staff at any time of the day or night if he has problems and can be admitted for a short rest as necessary (the team try to ensure that he is readmitted before things get too bad and there is a risk of him losing his accommodation). Had this support been forthcoming when he first lived in a flat a great deal of distress and disturbance, not to mention expense, could have been spared.

There has been one shift in resources from hospitals to supported community accommodation, there is now a need for another: from specialist sheltered housing support in independent accommodation. There are many ways in which such help can be provided and numerous research studies that demonstrate that intensive outreach support (like that described above) can be effective (Witheridge, 1989; Olfson, 1990; Ford and Repper, 1994; Ford et al., 1995). Despite this, the majority of people with serious ongoing mental health problems in the UK do not have access to this kind of help. In addition, where such help is available, it normally only becomes available after an unnecessarily large number of years of chaos, disruption and failure. Ensuring that people have help when things start to go wrong, rather than when they have broken down, is essential if people are not to have to waste an enormous amount of time and self-respect, and the consequent breakdown of relationships and roles, that such disruption almost invariably entails.

For many workers it is dispiriting to have to face running down and closing the brand new community facilities that have just been created, but such changes are essential if people with serious ongoing mental health problems are to live the lives that they wish to lead and if the negative consequences of their difficulties are to be minimized. Indeed, this was one of the fundamental principles of the residential services developed for old long-stay patients in Nottingham (Howat et al., 1988). In principle, everyone could live in their own place: there is no theoretical reason why a person could not receive the level of support they need, even if this meant as many as two staff being with them at all hours of the day or night. However, there are two practical reasons why this would not be possible. First, it would be exceedingly expensive and economies of scale will probably continue to dictate that those few people who need continuous supervision over long periods of time can only be provided with the support they require if they are grouped together. Second, there are some people whose behaviour is unlikely ever to become acceptable in ordinary community settings, especially those people whose violence, disturbance and sexually unacceptable behaviours cannot be decreased. Such people may continue to require an environment that can tolerate such behaviours (Shepherd *et al.*, 1994). However, it is important to remember that there are very few people who require such intensively staffed and tolerant environments: only a very small proportion of those currently living in staffed, group environments. Many of those who currently reside in such settings could manage in their own accommodation with the right type and degree of support. The support likely to be necessary has been documented by several authors (see Stein and Test, 1980; Lavender and Holloway, 1988; Ekdawi and Conning, 1994) and is likely to include the following.

- Rapidly available 'on-call' help at all hours of the day and night. This might be provided by closing a hostel or staffed setting and keeping the staff team who could work on a peripatetic basis, or by negotiating with housing authorities to provide a group of flats in one area so that they can be easily reached. This type of support would be much more flexible. If ordinary housing units were used, then this would allow a person to stop receiving support if they ceased to need it without having to move house. It would also allow a sensitive adjustment in level of support in response to changing needs. In any group setting a 'lowest common denominator' situation prevails: if one person needs staff presence 24 hours a day then everyone living there gets it whether they need/want it or not. Technology, such as mobile telephones and the type of on-call systems now available for elderly people, could be employed.
- A high level of support and help within a person's accommodation or close at hand. It is not necessary for people to be able to look after their flat, feed themselves or manage their own money and medication in order to have their own home. If cleaners were supplied, if meals were provided at home, if washing was done, if someone came round with medication once or twice a day and helped the person to budget their money, pay bills, buy food, then many people could have a place of their own.
- Help to go to work and make use of leisure, education and social facilities. This could include the provision of transport and someone to go along with them. This need not be a member of staff: it would be entirely possible for other service users who have some idea about the difficulties people face to act as 'buddies'.
- Emotional support and help with problems as they arise, both through regular visits from a mental health worker (or 'buddy' service user) and on-call help.

For those who, despite a high level of support, remain unable to cope in their own accommodation there are many ways in which staffed accommodation can be rendered more like having a place of one's own. For example, we have seen highly staffed accommodation divided into individual flats. Nevertheless, where a person lives remains one part of their life: other areas are equally, if not more important.

NOT JUST SOMEWHERE TO SLEEP: THE IMPORTANCE OF WORK

Being 'in the community' is almost invariably defined in terms of where a person sleeps at night. This leads to the ludicrous situation that someone is defined as being 'in the community' if they live in a segregated sheltered setting outside hospital, spend all their time either in this accommodation or other segregated day facilities, and have no contacts or networks within the community in which they reside. Conversely, someone who lives on a hospital site but spends most of their waking hours outside (at work, in the pub, with friends) is considered to be hospitalized – 'not in the community' – even though they have extensive contacts and networks within the community.

A major challenge facing community care services is to move beyond a consideration of where a person lives, to the networks, contacts and roles that a person has within his or her communities. This means that there must be an increased focus on ways in which people can be supported in developing and maintaining social roles and relationships. As with accommodation, it is in a disabled individual's interests, and much more straightforward, to preserve roles, relationships and activities that they already have, rather than trying to regain these when they have been lost. When a person has lost their job because of mental health problems it is more difficult to get it back. When a person has lost contact with family and friends it is more difficult to re-establish these relationships. When a person has stopped engaging in leisure and spare time activities it is more difficult to restart these.

In work, social and leisure domains, there has been a tendency to establish, within community care services, specialist, segregated, mental health facilities and opportunities. As with specialist accommodation (hostels, supported houses) there are numerous day centres, drop-ins, social clubs and sheltered work facilities that are designed solely for people with mental health problems. The psychiatric hospital has been broken down into its component parts and scattered throughout communities and the individuals who use these services often remain almost as segregated as they were in the old institutions. Often their only contact with life outside is the journey from one specialist facility to another ... and walking along a street or travelling on a bus does not, for most people, constitute being a part of 'the community'. In general, we need to move away from the provision of special social, work and leisure opportunities to the provision of special support to ensure that the disabled person has access to ordinary facilities that already exist within communities.

The area of work is of particular significance in our society. It is the second question that we ask new people we meet (what is your name? what do you do?)

and an important way in which we define ourselves: in the words of Janice Galloway (1991, p. 11):

> This is my workplace. This is where I earn my definition, this is the place that tells me what I am.

Work affords us a social identity and status, a role and meaning in life. It provides social contacts and support, a sense of personal achievement, and structures time. It really is not possible to eat, drink or make love for eight hours a day (Rowland and Perkins, 1988). The presence and absence of work also have enormous implications for the mental health of anyone (Smith, 1985). In one London Borough, those who were unemployed were eight times more likely than those in work to be referred to psychiatric services (Perkins, 1994). For people who experience serious ongoing mental health problems work takes on even greater importance. The status and role it provides are critical to someone who only has the devalued identity of 'mental patient'. The contacts that work affords are vital for someone with very limited social networks. The distraction, predictability, and enforced activity of the work environment all provide conditions which are conducive to a decrease in cognitive and emotional problems and protect against secondary disabilities. The money which work brings is vital for those who experience the poverty of reliance on welfare benefits.

Despite its centrality in most people's lives, community care services have been notoriously unsuccessful in ensuring that those whom they serve have access to work: 85% of long term service users in the two London Boroughs are unemployed (Perkins and Arnold, 1994) and surveys of the same population show that a similar percentage want to work (Perkins, 1993). No one in the continuing community care services of another major UK city are employed (Repper and Perkins, 1994). Despite continued pleas for more attention to this area (see Bennett, 1980; Shepherd, 1984; Perkins and Rowland, 1990; Ekdawi and Conning, 1994) the majority of people with serious long term mental health problems remain unemployed.

In an age of high unemployment, work has become an increasingly scarce commodity amongst people with serious mental health problems. There are many people who entered long term care services in the early 1970s when unemployment began to increase: when the person who swept the leaves in the park also had to be a gardener, and the person who wiped tables in the café also had to serve food and work the till, many people whose employment was marginal lost their jobs. Similarly, many nationalized industries provided a tolerant work environment for people with mental health problems. We have now seen several 'privatization casualties': people with disabilities who have lost their employment as a consequence of the drive for efficiency and slimming down of the workforce that the privatization moves of the 1980s and 1990s necessitate.

It is important to distinguish between the concept of work and that of employment. Work is a purposeful activity that requires effort and discretion, has social significance and structures and organizes time, but it is not necessarily employment. Employment additionally refers to an economic exchange relationship between employer and employee (Hartley, 1980). As Shepherd (1984) argues:

> Work, even without the strict economic contingencies of labour and reward, will still fulfil many ... basic psychological and social needs.

Indeed, there are numerous types of work outside the mental health sphere – voluntary work, raising children, and so forth – that do not constitute paid employment but which have all the other attributes of a work role.

In general, psychiatric hospitals offered a great deal of segregated sheltered employment for their residents: initially maintaining the running of the hospital and its grounds, latterly in Industrial Units. In moves to community care, many of these work opportunities have not been reprovided elsewhere (House of Commons Social Services Committee, 1985). Prevailing divisions between health and social care often result in disputes about the responsibility for work provision: work, *par excellence*, spans this health/social divide by maintaining health (both mental and physical) and social connections, status and roles.

There are four additional factors in relation to work that have proved problematic for people with serious long term mental health problems. First, is the tendency to regard sheltered work as preparing people for employment. Many sheltered work facilities operate on a throughput model helping people to acquire the skills necessary to gain a job outside. Whilst there are some people for whom this can become a reality, even when employment was plentiful in the 1950s and 1960s, less than 40% of those attending industrial units were resettled in open employment (Wansborough, 1983). For a person with ongoing disabilities such a throughput model is as inappropriate in relation to work as it is in relation to other areas of life. If such people are to have access to work we must move away from a perspective of changing people to render them ready for work/employment. Instead, the perspective must be one of changing work/employment to render it ready for the people who need it. This can be done either in a sheltered setting or, preferably, by changing open employment so that socially disabled individuals can be accommodated. We will return to this point later.

Second, it is the fashion to argue that we are now living in a society of leisure. We have frequently heard mental health workers argue that we should not focus on work for disabled people but help them to use the 'leisure time' that their unemployment affords more productively. In our opinion this is a dangerously naïve position. Whilst there may be many people in the UK who are without work, this has not led to a situation in which a high status and value is accorded to unemployment. Thus, a person who is already devalued as a 'mental patient' is further devalued by their unemployment. If there is to be a move towards leisure being an acceptable way of life (and we have grave doubts whether this will occur) then is it reasonable to expect those who are amongst the most devalued and vulnerable to spearhead such developments? If a 'leisure society' is to develop then those who are in the more advantageous positions are in the best place to effect it. Indeed, it could be argued that, as work becomes a scarcer commodity, it should be reserved for those who most need it – people with serious mental health problems (Shepherd, 1984; Rowland and Perkins, 1988).

Third, there is also a naïvety on the part of many mental health workers concerning whether people with serious cognitive and emotional problems want to work. In surveys that we have conducted, over 80% of people with such difficulties wanted to work, yet mental health workers often argue that when it actually comes down to getting out of bed in the morning, many of these same people do not really want to go to work. This apparent conflict – a person both saying that they want to work and that they do not want to do so – is in fact a normal situation. The obligations involved in work are a central characteristic of it: we can do, or not do, leisure activities as we want, but work is something that we have to do (whether we want to or not) and it is this feature that provides the structure and purpose that work affords. Most people would say that we want to have a job, in general terms, but if asked whether they want to go to work when they wake up in the morning, or at the end of a bad day, we wonder how many of us would say yes? All of us can appear ambivalent about work – sometimes saying we want to do it, sometimes saying we do not – people with serious mental health problems are likely to be the same. However, one thing is clear: a work role is central to the lives of almost everyone in employment and its absence central for those who are unemployed.

Fourth, work training and provision for people with disabilities does not take into account the needs of those with the social disabilities resulting from ongoing mental health problems. There are various work schemes provided for disabled people, but these focus on the needs of those with physical or sensory limitations and learning disabilities. Rarely do such projects take into account the specific problems experienced by those who have ongoing mental health difficulties. For example, there is a tendency to demand that people turn up regularly and on time for work, get on with other workers and accept supervision. The specific disabilities associated with serious mental health problems can make a person seem unreliable, make it difficult for them to attend regularly and make relationships with other people problematic. This means that expectations of reliability and sociability explicitly exclude those with social disabilities. If work is to be rendered accessible to socially disabled people, then it must be tailored to their specific needs: cater for such problems as erratic attendance, attentional deficits and social problems in the same way as might occur for sight and mobility limitations. In this context, it is important to note that the amount of time that someone with social disabilities is absent from work may not differ from that of someone without such disabilities, but the pattern of this absenteeism may be different. Perkins (1991b) showed that (with the exception of the most erratic attenders), during a three-month period, the amount of time off amongst workers at a hospital-based industrial unit did not differ from that of nurses in a ward at the same hospital. However, the industrial unit workers worked significantly fewer complete weeks in the period. The data indicated that industrial unit workers tended to take the odd day off here and there, whilst nurses tended to be off for longer blocks of time.

Clearly, this relative lack of predictability in attendance may cause problems in a work setting, but there are ways in which adaptations such as flexible rostering, flexitime, changed work patterns and support services could be used to render work, or preferably employment, accessible for someone with these difficulties. For example, the data from the above study indicated that it would have been possible to compensate for the relatively unreliable attendance of each worker. Each of this particularly disabled group was off an average of one day per week, but the number of people who attended work each day was remarkably stable: a 20% increase in the workforce would have easily compensated for the absenteeism. It should be noted that this is a lower percentage than the 25% used to augment nursing staff numbers to cover absenteeism (holidays, study leave and sickness).

This type of accommodation of social disability has been used in various projects in the USA to enable people with these disabilities to engage in open employment. For example, we have seen schemes where jobs are held not by one individual but by a mental health service (Perkins, 1993). This service then guarantees that the job will be completed. A group of people may share the job, or a job coach may help the person to do it and work in their place if they are not able to attend. In this way the employer is happy because they get the work done and seriously disabled people have an opportunity of employment. Other supports and adaptations to ensure access might include the availability of a mental health worker to provide help and resolve problems that arise both on a planned and an 'on-call' basis during work hours, help to get to work (the provision of transport or an early morning call) and the modifications to the work environment to minimize the difficulties a person has in working alongside others.

In an age of high unemployment, it should not be forgotten that the health service is the UK's largest employer. Within mental health services there are numerous employment opportunities that could be made available to people with mental health problems. In the service in which one of us works we have several seriously socially disabled people working in ordinary posts in the portering and other non-clinical areas. Further, the specific skills and experience of people with mental health problems have been used to help others with similar difficulties. At the time of writing there are service users employed to run groups for other service users, to assist in the running of a clinic where those prescribed the anti-psychotic drug, clozapine, come to have their blood tests, and in the running of recreational activities. Building on this success, a supported employment scheme has recently been started to enable people with serious mental health problems to work in mental health teams in ordinary mental health support worker and nursing assistant jobs. This is based on the similar highly successful scheme that has been operating in Colorado, USA, for many years (Sherman and Porter, 1991).

As with accommodation and leisure/social activities, in the area of work we need to move away from a model of providing special sheltered work (at very low pay) for people with mental health problems. The challenge is to support people in ordinary, open employment rather than sheltered workshops. However, there are likely to be some people who, despite high levels of support, will not be able to sustain open employment. For these people, some form of sheltered work may continue to be necessary. However, such sheltered work can still ensure maximum community integration by being designed to ensure contact with non-disabled people. This can be achieved where a product is sold to the public or where a service is performed for others (gardening etc.).

It is often assumed that providing work opportunities requires large-scale initiatives that are beyond the scope of individual mental health workers. This does not have to be the case. We have seen a great many small-scale enterprises affording a valuable service that have been established by individual mental workers in the course of their other responsibilities. For example, car-washing services, second-hand clothes shops and recycling projects. Indeed, it may be useful to set up a kind of 'small business bureau' to assist in the establishment of such small-scale enterprises by providing such things as secretarial and office back-up and small amounts of start-up funding.

In terms of accommodation, work, leisure and social relationships, a shift in focus is necessary: a move away from this specialist, segregated community facilities towards the support in ordinary facilities, activities and roles. Although at present, most of those who would formerly have spent their lives in psychiatric institutions are now physically located outside hospital, the challenge is to move from a physical presence to a valued role: to enable people with mental health problems to become a part of the communities in which they live and to participate in those communities as valued citizens.

In working towards this end, the aim is not to change individuals so that they can 'fit in' but to change communities so that they are accessible and can accommodate disabled individuals. The mass re-education of communities is almost certainly a non-starter, but a process of attrition can and does work. This means starting at the level of specific leisure, social, work and accommodation facilities and helping individual people to have access and participate. This is a task in which all can become involved. On a small scale, mental health workers (or indeed other service users) can facilitate access to pubs, clubs, bingo halls, sports facilities ... the list is almost endless. And people with mental health problems are their own best advocates. The presence of someone with disabilities in one's midst is a far more effective way of changing attitudes and facilitating access than is a lecture by a mental health professional. Essentially, the challenge for community services is one of helping all of their disabled clients – not simply those who can 'pass' as non-disabled – to gain access to communities and enjoy their rights as citizens. However, rights of citizenship can rest uneasily with a mental health worker's 'duty of care'.

DUTY OF CARE AND THE RIGHTS OF DISABLED INDIVIDUALS

Throughout mental health services runs an assumption that it is the duty of workers to provide vulnerable individuals with the help and support that they need. The right-wing political climate may have dented this premise with increased emphasis on individual freedom, however, amongst most of the population, the ideology on which the 'welfare state' was founded remains strong: we must 'do something' to help those who cannot help themselves. At first sight such desires seem entirely laudable but, on more detailed consideration, numerous problems emerge.

To begin at the level of individual support, a mental health professional's 'duty of care' rests upon an understanding of a disabled individual's needs. We have already discussed the many ways in which the concept of need is problematic, but in terms of the present discussion 'who defines a need?' is the critical question. In practice, needs are defined by mental health workers on the basis of information they may collect from a variety of sources: their own observations and assessments, those involved with the individual (family, friends, other professional contacts such as General Practitioners and other non-NHS mental health facilities and personnel), and the person him/herself. Needs identified from these sources may be the same, but such coincidence is unlikely as staff, family/friends and the individual him/herself have different interests and concerns. For example, if someone plays their record player late into the night it is unlikely to represent problems to them, but it may to others with whom the person lives. Because of this frequent lack of concordance in that which is defined as a need, choices have to be made about whose definition to adopt. It is not surprising that needs identified by staff are more likely to be reflected in care plans than are those identified by the client who is the recipient of the care (Perkins and Fisher, 1995). Even if equal weight were attached to the views of each of the interested parties, it would still be the case that some of the needs addressed would not be considered needs by the individual concerned.

Inherent in this type of system is the existence of a plan that only in part reflects the expressed concerns of the client. If mental health workers make decisions about what a person needs then they are assuming that they know better than the client: that they have a right to make decisions for people because they are not capable of making such decisions for themselves. Mental health workers justify doing this by recourse to their 'duty of care' – a duty to look after those who cannot look after themselves – but immediately the client's civil rights are infringed in a way that workers themselves would almost certainly resent if it happened to them.

It is hard to stand by and watch someone do something that we believe to be profoundly detrimental to them: allow someone to live in squalor or risk physical assault. Clearly, any society imposes limits on the behaviour of its citizens: the central issue is whether different limits should be imposed upon those who are disabled by serious mental health problems. At present, those with such problems are not only limited by the laws that apply to everyone else but also by the special laws just for them enshrined in mental health legislation. There may be many justifications for this unequal position, but it nevertheless means that those with cognitive and emotional problems are treated differently: do not have the rights of other citizens. There is a conflict between care and protection, and individual rights.

This conflict is not one to which there are easy answers and the situation that prevails is an ever changing compromise between individual rights and care and protection of the individual and of others. In the UK, mental health legislation up to the 1983 Mental Health Act, generally moved in the direction of increasing individual rights, but more recently there has been a swing in the other direction of greater powers to control the behaviour of those living outside hospital. As we have already argued, it is not only the legislative framework that is of concern: there are many ways in which mental health services exercise power over those whom they serve, and where conflicts between individual rights and duty of care arise. In essence, if someone does not do what mental health workers think is best for them there is often an assumption that they must be coerced into doing it 'for their own good'. Whilst this may be done from the most honourable and caring of motives, it nevertheless devalues the opinions of those who have serious mental health problems and denies their rights. Society will undoubtedly deem some behaviours to be unacceptable, but it is our opinion that we need, both individually and collectively, to move away from a perspective based on 'duty of care' to one predicated on individual rights to care and support.

This would mean a radical change. Instead of starting from a premise based on the **duty of professionals** we would move to one based on the **rights of people with serious mental health problems**. Everyone with such difficulties has a right to information, help, support, treatment and where necessary, shelter ... but they also have the right to refuse these things if they do not want them or they are not to their liking.

Overview: Ensuring access

Throughout this book we have argued that the primary aim of mental health services for people who are seriously disabled by ongoing cognitive and emotional problems must be to ensure that they have access to roles, relationships and activities in the communities of their choice, and can, as far as possible, live the lives that they choose. The myths and stigma associated with serious mental health problems make many people unwelcoming of those with such difficulties: it is for services to ensure that these barriers are broken down. Numerous difficulties can prevent disabled people availing themselves of the opportunities that are their right: it is for services to provide that help and support which is necessary to circumvent these problems. However, if it is to be of any value at all, the support and help provided must be accessible to the disabled individual.

If a person declines to avail themselves of support, then the most important question is 'Why is this service unacceptable to them?' There are many aspects of services that are unpleasant – ranging from the physical structures to the way in which users are treated. How many mental health workers would choose to enter one of the wards or day services in which they work? How many of them can honestly say that they treat clients in the respectful and dignified manner which they themselves would expect? How many would accept treatment without knowing the pros and cons of all the options available?

We need to move away from a position that alternatively asserts that 'If a person does not accept what is good for them, we have a duty to ensure that they get it' and 'If a person refuses what we have to offer them it is their problem not ours'. Instead, if a person does not accept the support available then they must have found it unacceptable. Either they have been offered the wrong thing or the right thing has been offered in the wrong way. From this perspective the onus is on mental health workers and services to change what they do, rather than on the person to change their mind and accept what services think they need. If we are unsure how to change what we do, then would it not be a good idea to ask the client?

There will be times when it is hard to adhere to such a principle: when someone who is profoundly depressed wants to kill themselves, when someone who is acutely psychotic becomes a danger to their family and friends. The ethics of such situations can, and will, be hotly debated. We have already discussed how it is possible to agree with a person, when they are not in a crisis, what they would like to happen when crises do occur. Clearly, this would not cover the first crisis that a person has, but it would enable them to decide what happens in subsequent ones. For the most part, people with serious ongoing mental health problems are able to make judgements and decisions most of the time. If such people are to be valued members of communities then they must have the same rights as others. This includes the right to help and support of a type, and in a manner, that is acceptable to them, rather than being forced against their will to accept that which they do not want.

Of course, increasing the rights of clients can be threatening to mental health workers. Threatening because they challenge the power that mental health services have long assumed over those they purport to serve. Threatening because they challenge the assumed right of professionals to know what is best for a person. Threatening because they place the onus on the mental health worker to provide what the individual wants. It is the responsibility of those who provide services if people who need support refuse that which is offered: it is their duty to render support more accessible and acceptable.

There are many challenges facing services for people who are disabled by ongoing mental health problems. These challenges cannot be left to 'someone else' to deal with and shortage of funding cannot be blamed for all ills. The acceptability and accessibility of services applies at all levels, from planning to the delivery of support by individual workers. It is the interactions and relationships with individual workers that most profoundly influence a person's experience of the services they receive. If people are infantilized and devalued within services then it is unlikely that they will readily accept the opinions of mental health workers or the support they offer. If we are truly to be allies, we must listen to those who use services, hear what they have to say, tailor what we offer accordingly (or explain why we are unable to meet their reasonable requests when we cannot) and always treat everyone, no matter how disabled, in the courteous and respectful manner that everyone has a right to expect. We need to look particularly at the views of those groups whom services most obviously fail and use the lessons that such an examination can afford to improve services for everyone with serious ongoing problems.

Even the best community services available at the time of writing are a long way from being perfect, or even really adequate. No one can rest on their laurels, but all workers at all levels have very real powers to change the services that are offered and users' experience of them. Like any other citizens, people who are disabled by serious ongoing mental health problems have a right of access to activities, roles and relationships in the communities relevant to them ... and to the support they need to avail themselves of these opportunities.

Increasingly powerful service user/survivor movements throughout the world are asserting their rights and beginning to provide alternatives to traditional psychiatric models and practice. If services cannot change they will become increasingly stigmatized and marginalized by those people with serious ongoing mental health problems who use them. Specialist mental health services must rise to the challenge of providing genuinely acceptable and accessible support that accord with the wants and wishes of those whom they serve.

References

Allen, H., Halperin, J. and Friend, R. (1985) Removal and diversion tactics and the control of auditory hallucinations. *Behaviour, Research and Therapy*, **23**, 601–5.

Allyon, T. and Azrin, N.H. (1968) *The Token Economy: A Motivational System for Therapy and Rehabilitation*, Appleton-Century-Crofts, New York.

Ambelas, A. (1979) Psychologically stressful events and the precipitation of manic episodes. *British Journal of Psychiatry*, **150**, 235–40.

Ambelas, A. (1987) Life events and mania – a special relationship? *British Journal of Psychiatry*, **150**, 235–40.

Anthony, L.A. (1977) Psychological rehabilitation – a concept of need in a method. *American Psychologist*, **1977**, 658–62.

Anthony, L.A. (1979) The rehabilitation approach to diagnosis. *New Directions in Mental Health Services*, **2**, 25–36.

Anthony, L.A. and Margules, A. (1974) Toward improving the efficacy of psychiatric rehabilitation: A skills training approach. *Rehabiliation Psychology*, **21**, 101–5.

Audit Commission (1994) *Finding a Place: A Review of Mental Health Services for Adults*, HMSO, London.

Bachrach, L.L. (1982) Foreword in R.H. Lamb (ed.), *Treating the Long-term Mentally Ill*, Jossey-Bass, San Francisco.

Bachrach, L.L. (1985) Chronically mentally ill women: Emergence and legitimation of programme issues. *Hospital and Community Psychiatry*, **36**, 1063–9.

Bachrach, L.L. (1988) Defining mental illness: A concept paper. *Hospital and Community Psychiatry*, **38**, 383–8.

Bachrach, L.L. (1989) The legacy of model programmes. *Hospital and Community Psychiatry*, **40**, 234–5.

Barker, P. (1992) Psychiatric nursing, in *Clinical Supervision and Mentorship in Nursing* (eds T. Butterworth and J. Faugier), Chapman & Hall, London.

Barton, R. (1959) *Institutional Neurosis*, Wright, Bristol.

Bateson, G., Jackson, D.D., Haley, J. *et al.* (1956) Toward a communication theory of schizophrenia. *Behavioural Science*, **1**, 251–64.

Beels, C.C., Gutwirth, L., Berkeley, J. *et al.* (1984) Measurement of social support in schizophrenia. *Schizophrenia Bulletin*, **10**, 399–411.

Bellack, A.S. (1986) Schizophrenia: Behaviour therapy's forgotten child. *Behaviour Therapy*, **17**, 249–53.

Bender, C.C. and Pilling, S. (1985) A study of the variables associated with under-attendance at a psychiatric day centre. *Psychological Medicine*, **15**, 395–401.

Bennett, D. (1978) Social forms of psychiatric treatment, in *Schizophrenia: Toward a New Synthesis* (ed. J.K. Wing), Academic Press, London.

Bennett, D. (1980) The chronic psychiatric patient today. *Journal of the Royal Society of Medicine*, **73**, 301–3.

Bentall, R.P., Jackson, H.F. and Pilgrim, D. (1988) Abandoning the concept of schizophrenia: Some implications of the validity arguments of psychological research into psychotic phenomena. *British Journal of Clinical Psychology*, **27**, 303–24.

Bentall, R.P., Claridge, G.S. and Slade, P. (1989) The multi-dimensional nature of schizotype traits: A factor analysis with normal subjects. *British Journal of Clinical Psychology*, **28**, 363–75.

Berke, J.H. (1979) *I Haven't Had To Go Mad Here*. Pelican, Harmondsworth.

Birch, A. (1983) *What Chance Have We Got?* MIND, London.

Birchwood, M. and Tarrier, N. (eds) (1992) *Innovations in the Psychological Management of Schizophrenia*. Wiley, Chichester.

Birchwood, M., Macmillan, F. and Smith, J. (1992) Early intervention, in *Innovations in the Psychological Management of Schizophrenia* (eds M. Birchwood and N. Tarrier), Wiley, Chichester.

Birley, J. (1991) Schizophrenia: The problems of handicap, in *Community Psychiatry* (eds D. Bennett and H. Freeman), Churchill Livingstone, London.

Birley, J. (1995) Paper given at Good Practices in Community Nursing Conference: Psychosocial Interventions in People with Serious and Enduring Mental Health Problems, 10 May 1995, Manchester University.

Blumhagen, D.W. (1981) On the nature of explanatory models. *Culture, Medicine and Psychiatry*, **5**, 337–40.

Boud, D., Keogh, R. and Walker, D. (1985) *Reflection: Turning Experience into Learning*, Kogan Page, London.

Boydell, K.M., Trainor, J.N. and Pierri, A.M. (1989) The effect of group homes for the mentally ill on residential property values. *Hospital and Community Psychiatry*, **40**, 957–8.

Boyle, M. (1990) *Schizophrenia: A Scientific Delusion?* Routledge, London.

Brett-Jones, J., Garety, P. and Hemsley, D. (1987) Measuring delusional experiences: A method and its application. *British Journal of Clinical Psychology*, **26**, 257–65.

Brewin, C.R., Wing, J.K., Mangen, S.P. *et al.* (1987) Principles and practice of measuring needs in the long-term mentally ill: The MRC needs for care assessment. *Psychological Medicine*, **17**, 971–81.

Brewin, C.R., Wing, J.K., Mangen, S.P. *et al.* (1988) Needs for care among the long-term mentally ill: A report from the Camberwell High Contact Survey. *Psychological Medicine*, **18**, 457–68.

Brooker, C.G.D. (1990) A description of clients nursed by community psychiatric nurses whilst attending English National Board Course No. 811: Clarification of current role. *Journal of Advanced Nursing*, **15**, 155–6.

Brooker, C.G.D., Falloon, I., Butterworth, T., *et al.* (1994) The outcome of training CPNs to deliver psychosocial intervention. *British Journal of Psychiatry*, **165**, 122–30.

Brown G. (1985) The discovery of expressed emotion: Induction or deduction?, in *Expressed Emotion in Families* (eds J. Leff and C. Vaughn), Guildford Press, New York.

Brown, G.W. and Birley, J.L.T. (1968) Crises and life changes and the onset of schizophrenia. *Journal of Health and Social Behaviour*, **9**, 203–14.

Brown, G.W. and Harris, T. (1978) *Social Origins of Depression*, Tavistock, London.

Brown, G., Carstairs, G. and Topping, G. (1958) Post hospital adjustment of chronic mental patients. *Lancet*, **2**, 685–9.

Brown, G.W., Bone, M., Dalison, M. and Wing, J.K. (1966) *Schizophrenia and Social Care*, Oxford University Press, Oxford.

Burnard, P. (1988) Equality and Meaning: Issues in the interpersonal relationship. *Community Psychiatric Nursing Journal*, **December**, 17–21.

Bynon, R. (1994) Personal Communication, MACA (Mental After Care Association).

Chadwick, P.D.J. and Lowe, C.F. (1990) Measurement and modification of delusional beliefs. *Journal of Consulting and Clinical Psychology*, **58**, 225–32.

Chamberlin, J. (1977) *On Our Own*, MIND Publications, London (1988 edition).

Chesler, P. (1972) *Women and Madness*, Avon Books, New York.

Christie-Brown, J.R.W., Ebringer, L. and Freedman, K.S. (1977) A survey of long-stay psychiatric population: Implications for community services. *Psychological Medicine*, **7**, 113–26.

Ciompi L. (1988) Learning from outcome studies: Towards a comprehensive biological–psychosocial understanding of schizophrenia. *Schizophrenia Research*, **1**, 373 84.

Clifford, P. (1989) *Evaluating the Closure of Cane Hill Hospital: Plans for Residential Services and the Long-Stay Population*, National Unit for Psychiatric Research and Development, London.

Coid, J.W. (1988) Mentally abnormal prisoners on remand. 1. Accepted or rejected by the NHS? *British Medical Journal*, **296**, 1779–82.

Confederation of Indian Organisations (1992) *A Cry for Change*, CIO, London.

Creer, C., Sturt, E. and Wykes, T. (1982) The role of relatives, in *Long Term Community Care: Experience in a London Borough* (ed. J.K. Wing), Psychological Monograph Supplement 2, 29–39.

David, A.S. (1990) Insight and Psychosis. *British Journal of Psychiatry*, **157**, 355–8.

Day, R., Neilson, J.A. and Korten, A. (1987) Stressful life events preceding the acute onset of schizophrenia: A cross-national study from the World Health Organisation. *Culture, Medicine and Society*, **11**, 123–205.

Day, J., Wood, G., Dewey, M., and Bentall, R.P. (1995) A self-rating scale for measuring side effects: Validation in a group of schizophrenic patients. *British Journal of Psychiatry* (in press).

Dear, M. (1990) *Gaining Community Acceptance*, The Robin Wood Johnson Foundation, Princeton.

Dear, M. (1992) Understanding and overcoming the NIMBY syndrome. *Journal of the American Planning Association*, **58**, 288–300.

Dear, M. and Gleeson, B. (1991) Community attitudes towards the homeless. *Urban Geography*, **12**, 155–76.

Dear, M. and Taylor, S.M (1982) *Not on Our Street: Community Attitudes to Mental Health Care*, Pion, London.

Dear, M. and Wolch, J. (1987) *Landscapes of Despair: From Institutionalisation to Homelessness,* Princeton University Press, Princeton.

Deegan, P.E. (1993) Recovering our sense of value after being labelled. *Journal of Psychosocial Nursing,* **31,** 7–11.

Department of Health and Social Services (1975) *Better Services for the Mentally Ill,* HMSO, London.

Dincin, J. (1993) Ending stigma and discrimination begins at home. *Hospital and Community Psychiatry,* **44,** 309.

Dittman, J. (1990) Disease consciousness and coping strategies of patients with schizophrenic psychosis. *Acta Psychiatrica Scandanavica,* **82,** 318–22.

DOH (1983) *The Mental Health Act,* HMSO, London.

DOH (1989a) *Caring for People: Community Care into the Next Decade and Beyond,* London, HMSO.

DOH (1989b) HC(89)5 *Discharge of Patients from Hospital,* HMSO, London.

DOH (1990a) *NHS and Community Care Act,* HMSO, London.

DOH (1990b) HC(90)23 *The Care Programme Approach for People with a Mental Illness,* HMSO, London.

DOH (1990c) HC(90)24 *Specific Grant for the Development of Social Services for People with a Mental Illness,* HMSO, London.

DOH (1991) *Implementing Community Care,* HMSO, London.

DOH (1992) *Health of the Nation,* HMSO, London.

DOH/Home Office (1993a) *Review of Health and Socal Services for Mentally Disordered Offenders and Others Requiring Similar Services: Volume 5, Special Issues and Differing Needs,* HMSO, London.

DOH (1993b) *Legal Powers on the Care of Mentally Ill People in the Community: Report of the Internal Review,* HMSO, London.

DOH (1993c) *Vision for the Future,* HMSO, London.

DOH (1994a) *Working in Partnership,* HMSO, London.

DOH (1994b) *Health of the Nation Key Area Handbook: Mental Illness,* 2nd edn, HMSO, London.

Done, D.J., Frith, C.D. and Owens, D.C. (1986) Reducing persistent auditory hallucinations by wearing an ear plug. *British Journal of Clinical Psychology,* **25,** 151–2.

Duldt, B.W., Giffin, K and Patton, B.R. (1983) *Interpersonal Communication in Nursing: A Humanistic Approach,* F.A. Davis, Philadelphia.

Eisenbruch, M. (1990) Classification of natural and supernatural causes of mental distress. *Journal of Nervous and Mental Disease,* **178,** 712–19.

Ekdawi, M. and Conning, A. (1994) *Psychiatric Rehabilitation: A Practical Guide,* Chapman & Hall, London.

Estroff, S. (1993) Community Mental Health Services: Extinct, Endangered or Evolving? Paper presented at the conference Mental Health Practices in the Nineties – Changes and Challenges, Silver Springs, Maryland, USA.

Fadden, G., Bebbington, P. and Kuipers, L. (1987) The burden of care: Impact of functional psychiatric illness on the patient's family. *British Journal of Psychiatry,* **164** (suppl. 23), 71–6.

Falco, K.L. (1991) *Psychotherapy with Lesbian Clients: Theory into Practice,* Brunner/Mazel, New York.

Falloon, R.H. and Fadden, G. (1993) *Integrated Mental Health Care: A Comprehensive Community Based Approach,* Cambridge University Press, Cambridge.

Falloon, I., Boyd, J. and McGill, C. (1982) Family management in the prevention of exacerbations of schizophrenia: A controlled study. *New England Journal of Medicine*, **306**, 437–440.

Falloon, I., Boyd, J. and McGill, C. (1984) *Family Care of Schizophrenia*, Guildford Press, New York.

Falloon, I., Boyd, J. and McGill, C. *et al.* (1985) Family management in the prevention of morbidity of schizophrenia. *Archives of General Psychiatry*, **34**, 171–84.

Fernando, S. (1991) *Mental Health, Race and Culture*, MIND/Macmillan, London.

Fernando, S. (1995) Study did not deal with 'Category fallacy'. *British Medical Journal*, **310**, 331–32.

Fishe, M. (1984) *Mental Health Social Work Observed*, National Institute of Social Services Library, No. 45.

Ford, R. and Repper, J. (1994) Taking responsibility for care. *Nursing Times*, **90**, 54–7.

Ford, M., Goddard, C. and Lansdallwelfare, R. (1987) The dismantling of the mental hospital? Glenside Hospital Surveys 1960–1985. *British Journal of Psychiatry*, **151**, 479–85.

Ford, R., Beadsmoore, A., Ryan, P. *et al.* (1995) Providing the safety net: Case management for people with a serious mental illness. *Journal of Mental Health*, **1**, 91–9.

Francis, E., David, J., Johnson, N. *et al.* (1989) Black people and psychiatry in the UK: An alternative to institutional care. *Psychiatric Bulletin*, **13**, 482–5.

Frith, C. (1979) Consciousness, information processing and schizophrenia. *British Journal of Psychiatry*, **134**, 333–40.

Galloway, J. (1991) *The Trick is to Keep Breathing*, Minerva, London.

Gelberg, L. and Linn, L. (1988) Social and physical health of homeless adults previously treated for mental health problems. *Hospital and Community Psychiatry*, **39**, 510–16.

Gilman, S. (1987) Alternatives to open employment in the community. *British Journal of Occupational Therapy*, **50**, 158–60.

Glass, J.M. (1989) *Private Terror/Public Life: Psychosis and the Politics of Community*, Cornell University Press, Ithaca.

Goffman, E. (1961) *Asylums*, Pelican, Harmondsworth.

Goldman, H. (1980) Mental illness and family burden: A public health perspective. *Hospital and Community Psychiatry*, **33**, 557–9.

Good Practices in Mental Health/European Regional Council World Federation for Mental Health (1994) *Women and Mental Health: An Information Pack of Mental Health Services for Women in the U.K.*, GPMH, London.

Gorman, J. (1992) *Out of the Shadows*, MIND, London.

Gove, W.L. (1975) Labelling mental illness: A critique, in *The Labelling of Deviance* (ed. W.L. Gove), Wiley, New York.

Gripp, R.F. and Magaro, P.A. (1974) The token economy program in the psychiatric hospital: A review and analysis. *Behaviour Research and Therapy*, **135**, 1193–7.

Hall, P., Brockington, I.F., Levings, J. *et al.* (1993) A comparison of responses to the mentally ill in two communities. *British Journal of Psychiatry*, **162**, 99–108.

Harding, C.M., Brooks, C.W., Ashikaga, T. *et al.* (1978) The Vermont longitudinal study of persons with severe mental illness II: Long-term outcome of subjects who once met the DSM III criteria for schizophrenia. *American Journal of Psychiatry*, **144**, 727–34.

Harrison, G., Owens, D., Holton A. *et al.* (1988) A prospective study of severe mental disorder in Afro-Caribbean patients. *Psychological Medicine*, **18**, 643–57.

Hartley, J.F. (1980) The impact of unemployment upon the self esteem of managers. *Journal of Occupational Psychology*, **53**, 145–7.

Hatfield, A.B. (1987) The expressed emotion theory: Why families object. *Hospital and Community Psychiatry*, **38**, 341.

Hatfield, A. (1989) Patient's accounts of stress and coping in schizophrenia. *Hospital and Community Psychiatry*, **40**, 137–44.

Helman, C. (1984) *Culture Health and Illness*, Wright, Bristol.

Hemsley, D. (1987) An experimental psychological model of schizophrenia, in *Search for the Causes of Schizophrenia* (eds H. Hafner, W.F. Galtaz and W. Janzavick), Springer-Verlag, Heidelberg.

Hirsch, S. (Chair) (1992) Facilities and Services for the Mentally Ill with Persisting Severe Disabilities. Working Party Report on Behalf of the Royal College of Psychiatrists.

Hogarty, G., Anderson, C., Reiss, D. and Kornblith, S. (1986) Family psycho-education, social skills training and maintenance chemotherapy in the aftercare of schizophrenia. *Archives of General Psychiatry*, **43**, 633–42.

Hoult, J. (1986) Community care of the acutely mentally ill. *British Journal of Psychiatry*, **149**, 137–44.

House of Commons Social Services Committee (1985) *Community Care with Special Reference to Mentally Ill and Mentally Handicapped People*, Second report from the Social Services Committee, HMSO, London.

Howat, J., Bates, P., Pidgeon, J. *et al.* (1988) The development of residential services in the community, in *Community Care in Practice: Services for the Continuing Care Client* (eds A. Lavender and F. Holloway), Wiley, Chichester.

Howe, G. (1994) *Schizophrenia: A Needs Based Approach*, Jessica Kingsley, London.

Huq, S.F., Garety, P. and Hemsley, D. (1988) Probabilistic judgements in deluded and non-deluded subjects. *Quarterly Journal of Experimental Psychology*, **40A**, 801–2.

Hustig, H.H., Tran, D.B., Hafner, R.J. *et al.* (1990) The effect of headphone music on persistent auditory hallucinations. *Behavioural Psychotherapy*, **18**, 273–82.

Ineichen, B., Harrison, G. and Morgan, H.G. (1984) Psychiatric hospital admissions in Bristol: I. Geographic and ethnic factors. *British Journal of Psychiatry*, **145**, 600–4.

Jacobs, H.E., Wissusik, D., Collier, R. *et al.* (1992) Correlations between psychiatric disabilities and vocational outcome. *Hospital and Community Psychiatry*, **43**, 365–9.

Johnson, B. (1995) Therapeutic attitudes: The clients' perception. Diploma Dissertation, Department of Nursing and Midwifery Studies, Nottingham University.

Johnstone, E.C., Owens, D.G.C., Gold, A., Crow, T.J. and Macmillan, J.F. (1984) Schizophrenic patients discharged from hospital – a follow-up study. *British Journal of Psychiatry*, **145**, 586–90.

Johnstone, L. (1989) *Users and Abusers of Psychiatry: A Critical Look at Traditional Psychiatric Practice*, Routledge, London.

Kazdin, A.E. (1978) *The Token Economy*, Plenum Press, New York.

King, R., Raynes, N. and Tizard, J. (1971) *Patterns of Residential Care*, Routledge, London.

King, M., Coker, E., Leavey, G. *et al.* (1994) Incidence of psychotic illness in London: Comparison of ethnic groups. *British Medical Journal*, **309**, 1115–19.

Kingdon, D.G. (1992) Interprofessional collaboration in mental health. *Journal of Interprofessional Care*, **6**, 141–6.

Kings Fund Centre (1995) *Clinical Supervision in Practice*, BEBC, Dorset.

Kitzinger, C. (1990) Heterosexism in psychology. *The Psychologist*, **September**, 391–2.

Kitzinger, C. and Perkins, R.E. (1993) *Changing Our Minds: Lesbian Feminism and Psychology*, Onlywomen Press, London.

Koran, M., Sox, H.C., Marton, K.I. *et al.* (1989) Medical evaluation of psychiatric patients 1: Results in a state mental health system. *Archives of General Psychiatry*, **46**, 733–40.

Kronemeyer, R. (1980) *Overcoming Homosexuality*, MacMillan, New York.

Kuipers, L. and Bebbington, P. (1988) Expressed emotion research in schizophrenia: Theoretical and clinical implications. *Psychological Medicine*, **18**, 893–909.

Lader, M. (1995) (Chair) *Guidelines for the Management of Schizophrenia*, Developed from a meeting of an independent working party, Lundbeck, London.

Laing, R.D. (1967) *The Politics of Experience and The Bird of Paradise*, Penguin, Harmondsworth.

Lavender, A. and Holloway, F. (eds) (1988) *Community Care in Practice: Services for the Continuing Care Client*, Wiley, Chichester.

Lazarus, R.S. and Folkman, S. (1984) Coping and adaptation, in *Handbook of Behavioural Medicine* (ed. E.D. Gentry), Guildford Press, London.

Leff, J.P. and Vaughn, C.E. (1985) *Expressed Emotion in Families*, Guildford Press, New York.

Leff, J., Berkowitz, R., Shavit, N. *et al.* (1989) A trial of family therapy v. A relatives group for schizophrenia. *British Journal of Psychiatry*, **154**, 58–66.

Leff, J., Kuipers, L., Berkowitz, R. *et al.* (1985) A controlled trial of social intervention in the families of schizophrenic patients: A two year follow up. *British Journal of Psychiatry*, **146**, 595–600.

Leventhal, H., Meyer, D. and Nerenz, D. (1980) The common-sense representation of illness and danger, in *Medical Psychology, Vol. 2* (ed. J. Rachman), Pergamon, New York.

Lewis, A. (1934) The psychopathology of insight. *British Journal of Medical Psychology*, **14**, 332–48.

Liberman, R.P., Mueser, K.T., Wallace, C.J. *et al.* (1986) Training skills in the psychiatrically disabled: Learning coping and competence. *Schizophrenia Bulletin*, **12**, 631–47.

Lindow, V. (1993) A service user's view, in *Mental Health Nursing: From First Principles to Professional Practice* (eds H. Wright and M. Giddey), Chapman & Hall, London.

Lowe, F. (1992) Cut off from care. *Community Care*, **August 27**.

Luckstead, A. and Coursey, R.D. (1995) Consumer perceptions of pressure and force in psychiatric treatment. *Hospital & Community Psychiatry*, **26**, 146–52.

Maden, A., Swinton, M. and Gunn, J. (1994) Psychiatric disorder in women serving a prison sentence. *British Journal of Psychiatry*, **164**, 44–54.

Mann, S. and Cree, W. (1976) 'New' long-stay patients: A national sample of 15 mental hospitals in England and Wales 1972–1973. *Psychological Medicine*, **6**, 603–16.

Marks, I.M., Connolly, J., Muijen, M. *et al.* (1994) Home based versus hospital based care for people with serious mental illness. *British Journal of Psychiatry*, **165**, 79–194.

Maslow, A. (1970) *Motivation and personality*, 2nd edn, Harper and Row, New York.

McGhie, A. and Chapman, J. (1961) Disorders of attention and perception in early schizophrenia. *British Journal of Medical Psychology*, **34**, 103–16.

McGrath, M.E. (1984) First person accounts: Where did I go? *Schizophrenia Bulletin*, **10**, 638–40.

Meltzer, D., Hale, S., Malik, S. *et al.* (1991) Community care for people with schizophrenia one year after discharge. *British Medical Journal*, **304**, 749–54.

Menn, A., Mosher, L. and Matthews, S. (1975) Soteria: Evaluation of a home-based treatment for schizophrenia. *American Journal of Orthopsychiatry*, **43**, 455–67.

Mental Health Foundation (1989) *Mental Health: The Fundamenal Facts*, Mental Health Foundation, London.

MIND (1994) *Policy on Black and Ethnic Minority People and Mental Health*, MIND Publications, London.

Moodley, P. and Perkins, R.E. (1991) Routes to care in an Inner London borough. *Social Psychiatry and Psychiatric Epidemiology*, **26**, 47–51.

Morley, S. (1987) Modification of auditory hallucinations: Experimental studies of head-phones and ear plugs. *Behavioural Psychotherapy*, **15**, 240–51.

Mowbray, C.T., Lanir, S. and Hulce, M. (eds) (1985) *Women and Mental Health*, Harrington Park Press, New York.

Muir, L. (1984) Teamwork, in *Social Work and Mental Health* (ed. M.R. Olsen), Tavistock, London.

National Schizophrenia Fellowship/Schizophrenia: A National Emergency (1988) *Mental Hospital Closures*, NSF, Surbiton, Surrey.

National Schizophrenia Fellowship (1995) *The Silent Partners*, NSF, London.

Nezu, A. and Ronan, G. (1985) Life stress, current problems, problem solving, and depressive symptoms: An integrative model. *Journal of Consulting and Clinical Psychology*, **53**, 693–9.

Norbeck, J.S., Chaftez, L. Skodol-Wilson, H. *et al.* (1991) Social support needs of family caregivers of psychiatric patients from three age groups. *Nursing Research*, **40**, 208–11.

Olfson, M. (1990) Assertive community treatment: An evaluation of experimental evidence. *Hospital and Community Psychiatry*, **41**, 634–41.

Patmore, C. and Weaver, T. (1991) Unnatural selection. *Health Services Journal*, **10th October**, 20–2.

Patterson, J.G. and Zderad, L.T. (1976) *Humanistic Nursing*, Wiley, New York.

Pembroke, L. (1991) Surviving psychiatry. *Nursing Times*, **87**, 30–2.

Perkins, R.E. (1991a) Oppression, inequality and invisible lesbians. *Feminism and Psychology*, **1**, 427–8.

Perkins, R.E. (1991b) Access to Work. Paper presented at the British Association for Behavioural Psychotherapy Annual National Conference, University of Oxford.

Perkins, R.E. (1992a) Working with socially disabled clients, in *Gender Issues in Clinical Psychology* (eds J. Ussher and P. Nicholson), Routledge, London.

Perkins, R.E. (1992b) Catherine is having a baby . . . *Feminism and Psychology*, **2**, 56–7.

Perkins, R.E. (1993) *Twelve States and Twenty Two Beds: A Tour of Innovative North American Community Care Services for People with Serious Ongoing Mental Health Problems*, Winston Churchill Travelling Fellowship Report, Pathfinder Community and Specialist Mental Health Services, London.

Perkins, R.E. (1994) *Report of the Wandsworth Mental Health Needs Assessment Project*, Wandsworth, Merton and Sutton Health Authority, London.

Perkins, R.E. (1995) Women, lesbians and community care, in *Planning Mental Health Services for Women: A Multiprofessional Handbook* (eds K. Abel, M. Buscewicz, S. Davison and E. Staples), Routledge, London.

Perkins, R.E. and Arnold, T. (1994) *1994 Long Term Care Case Register Report*, Pathfinder Mental Health Services NHS Trust, London.

Perkins, R.E. and Dilks, S. (1992) Worlds apart: Working with severely socially disabled people. *Journal of Mental Health*, **1**, 3–17.

Perkins, R.E. and Fisher, N. R. (1995a) Some ethnic groups may be more vulnerable to extremes of social deprivation. *British Medical Journal*, **310**, 332–3.

Perkins, R.E. and Fisher, N.R. (1995b) Beyond mere existence: The auditing of care plans. *Journal of Mental Health* (in press).

Perkins, R. E. and Greville, L. (1993) *Long-Term Care Register: Fourth Annual Report*, Pathfinder Mental Health Services NHS Trust, London.

Perkins, R.E. and Moodley, P. (1993a) Perceptions of problems in psychiatric inpatients: Denial, race and service usage. *Social Psychiatry and Psychiatric Epidemiology*, **28**, 114–19.

Perkins, R.E. and Moodley, P. (1993b) The arrogance of insight? *Psychiatric Bulletin*, **17**, 233–4.

Perkins, R.E. and Prince, S. (1993) *User's Views About Their Work Needs: A Survey of Rehabilitation and Continuing Care Clients*, Pathfinder Mental Health Services NHS Trust, London.

Perkins, R.E. and Rowland, L.A. (1990) Sex differences in service usage in long term psychiatric care: Are women adequately served? *British Journal of Psychiatry*, **158** (suppl. 10), 75–9.

Perkins, R.E., King, S. and Hollyman, J.A. (1989a) Resettlement of old long-stay psychiatric patients: The use of the private sector. *British Journal of Psychiatry*, **155**, 233–8.

Perkins, R.E., Fahey, K., Shinner, M. *et al.* (1989b) Barriers broken down. *Health Service Journal*, **99**, 1432–3.

Perkins, R.E., Hollyman, J.A., Boardman, C.J. *et al.* (1992) From long-stay patient to Sloane Ranger: Outcome of resettlement of 15 old long stay patients in warden-supervised accomodation for the elderly. *Journal of Mental Health*, **1**, 149–62.

Perring, C., Twigg, J. and Atkin, A. (1990) *Families Caring for Someone Diagnosed as Mentally Ill: The Literature Re-examined*, HMSO, London.

Podvoll, E. (1992) *The Seduction of Madness: A Compassionate Approach to Recovery at Home*, Century, London.

Rabkin, J.G., Muhlin, G. and Cohen, P.W. (1984) What the neighbours think: Attitudes towards local psychiatric facilities. *Community Mental Health Journal*, **20**, 304–12.

Rapp, C.A. and Wintersteen, R. (1989) The strengths model: Results from 12 demonstrations. *Psycho-Social Rehabilitation*, **13**, 23–32.

Repper, J. and Cooney, P. (1994) The policy context and organisation of care, in *Mental Health and Disorder*, 2nd edn (eds T. Thompson and P. Matthias), Baillière Tindall, London.

Repper, J. and Peacham, W. (1991) A suitable case for management. *Nursing Times*, **87**, 62–5.

Repper, J. and Perkins, R. (1994) Meeting the needs of neglected patients. *Nursing Standard*, **9**, 28–31.

Repper, J. and Perkins, R. (1995) Targeting a local service for the severely mentally ill: Implications for community psychiatric nurses, in *Community Psychiatric Nursing: A Research Perspective, Volume 3* (eds C. Brooker and E. White), Chapman & Hall, London.

Repper, J., Cooke, A. and Ford, R. (1994) How can nurses build trusting relationships with people who have severe and long term mental health problems? Experiences of case managers and their clients? *Journal of Advanced Nursing*, **19**, 1096–104.

Ritchie, J., Dick, D. and Lingham, R. (1994) *The Report of the Enquiry into the Care and Treatment of Christopher Clunis*, HMSO, London.

Rogers, K. (1957) The necessary and sufficient conditions of therapeutic personality change. *Journal of Counselling Psychology*, **21**, 95–103.

Rogers, A. and Faulkener, A. (1987) *A Place of Safety*, MIND Publications, London.

Romme, M.A.J., Honig, A., Hoorthorn, E.O. and Escher, A.D.M.C. (1992) Coping with hearing voices: An emancipatory approach. *British Journal of Psychiatry*, **161**, 99–103.

Rowland, L.A. and Perkins, R.E. (1988) You can't eat, drink and make love eight hours a day: The value of work in psychiatry. *Health Trends*, **20**, 75–9.

Ryan, P. (1979) Residential care for the mentally disabled, in *Community Care for the Mentally Disabled* (eds J.K. Wing and R. Olsen), Oxford University Press, Oxford.

Sandford, T. (1994) Users' perspectives of clinics providing depot phenothiazine treatments, in *Perspectives on Mental Health Nursing* (eds K. Gournay and T. Sandford), Scutari, London.

Sayce, L., Craig, T. and Boardman, A. (1991) The development of community mental health centres in the U.K. *Social Psychiatry and Psychiatric Epidemiology*, **26**, 14–20.

Scheff, T.J. (1967) *Mental Illness and Social Processes*, Harper and Row, London.

Scottish Association for Mental Health (1992) *Community Care and Consultation: A Report by the Scottish Mental Health Forum*, SAMH, Edinburgh.

Segal, S.P. and Aviram, U. (1978) *The Mentally-Ill in Community Based Sheltered Care*, Wiley, New York.

Segal, S.P., Baumohl, J. and Moyles, E.W. (1980) Neighbourhood types and community reaction to the mentally ill: A paradox of intensity. *Journal of Health and Social Behaviour*, **21**, 345–59.

Shepherd, G. (1977) Social skills training: The generalisation problem. *Behaviour Therapy*, **8**, 100–9.

Shepherd, G. (1978) Social skills training: The generalisation problem – some further data. *Behaviour Research and Therapy*, **116**, 287–8.

Shepherd, G.W. (1984) *Institutional Care and Rehabilitation*, Longman Applied Psychology, London.

Shepherd, G. (1988) Current Issues in Community Care. Report of the 2nd Annual Conference on the Rehabilitation of Psychiatric Patients and their Care in the Community, 13.12.88, The Association of Psychological Therapies, Leicester.

Shepherd, G. (1990) Case management. *Health Trends*, **22**, 59–61.

Shepherd, G., Murray, A. and Muijen, M. (1994) *Relative Values*, The Sainsbury Centre for Mental Health, London.

Sherman, P.S. and Porter, R. (1991) Mental health consumers as case management aides. *Hospital and Community Psychiatry*, **42**, 494–8.

Showalter E. (1987) *The Female Malady*, Virago, London.

Siegler, M. and Osmond, H. (1976) *Models of Madness, Models of Medicine*, Harper Colophon, New York.

Smith, R. (1985) Bitterness, shame, emptiness, waste: An introduction to unemployment and health, I. *British Medical Journal*, **291**, 1024–8.

Smith, J. and Birchwood, M. (1990) Relatives and patients as partners in the management of schizophrenia: The development of a service model. *British Journal of Psychiatry*, **156**, 654–60.

Solomon, P. (1983) Analysing opposition to community residential facilities for troubled adolescents. *Child Welfare*, **LXII**, 261–74.

Stein, L.I. and Test, M.A. (1980) Alternative to mental hospital I. Conceptual model, treatment programme and clinical evaluation. *Archives of General Psychiatry*, **37**, 392–7.

Stewart, W. (1985) *Counselling in Rehabilitation*, Croom Helm, London.

Strauss, J.S. (1994) The person with schizophrenia as a person II: Approaches to the subjective and complex. *British Journal of Psychiatry*, **164** (suppl. 23), 103–7.

Strauss, J.S., Rakfeldt, J., Harding, C.M. *et al.* (1989) Psychological and social aspects of negative symptoms. *British Journal of Psychiatry*, **155** (suppl. 7), 128–32.

Summers, F. and Hersch, S. (1983) Psychiatric chronicity and diagnosis. *Schizophrenia Bulletin*, **9**, 122–32.

Sundeen, R.A. and Fiske, S. (1982) Local resistance to community based care facilities. *Journal of Offender Counselling, Services and Rehabilitation*, **6**, 29–42.

Tarrier, N. (1992) Management and modification of residual psychotic symptoms, in *Innovations in the Psychological Management of Schizophrenia* (eds M. Birchwood and N. Tarrier), Wiley, Chichester.

Tarrier, N., Barrowclough, C., Vaughn, C. *et al.* (1988) The community management of schizophrenia: A controlled trial of behavioural intervention with families to reduce relapse. *British Journal of Psychiatry*, **153**, 532–42.

Taylor, K.E. and Perkins, R.E. (1991) Identity and coping with mental illness in long-stay psychiatric rehabilitation. *British Journal of Clinical Psychology*, **30**, 73–85.

Test, L. and Stein, M.A. (1978) Community treatment of the chronic patient: Research overview. *Schizophrenia Bulletin*, **4**, 350–64.

Timms, P.W. and Fry, A.H. (1989) Homelessness and mental illness. *Health Trends*, **21**, 71–2.

Torrey, E.F. (1983) *Surviving Schizophrenia: A Family Perspective*, Harper and Row, New York.

Vaughn, C. and Leff, J. (1976a) The measurement of expressed emotion in the families of schizophrenic patients. *British Journal of Social and Clinical Psychology*, **15**, 57–65.

Vaughn, C. and Leff, J. (1976b) The influence of family and social factors on the course of psychiatric illness. *British Journal of Psychiatry*, **129**, 125–37.

Waite, T. (1993) *Taken On Trust*, Hodder and Stoughton, London.

Wallace, M. (1989) A caring community? *Sunday Times Magazine*, **May 3rd**.

Wansborough, N. (1983) Sheltered industrial groups in the present setting. *Industrial Therapy*, **8**, 13–16.

Warden, A., Walsh, A. and Becker, S. (1990) *Sentenced to Live Within that Sickness: Mental Health, Social Security and Registered Homes*, Benefits Research Unit, Nottingham University.

Watts, F.N., Powell, G.E. and Austin, S.V. (1973) The modification of abnormal beliefs. *British Journal of Medical Psychology*, **46**, 359–63.

Weiss, M.G., Sharma, S.D., Gavr, R.K. *et al.* (1986) Traditional concepts of mental disorder among Indian psychiatric patients: Preliminary report of work in progress. *Social Science and Medicine*, **23**, 379–86.

Weller, M. (1989) Psychosis and destitution at Christmas 1985–1988. *Lancet*, **ii**, 1509–11.

Wells, K.B., Stewart, A., Hays, R.D. *et al.* (1989) The functioning and well being of depressed patients: Results from the medical outcomes study. *Journal of American Medical Association*, **262**, 914–19.

Wenocur, S. and Belcher, J. (1990) Strategies for overcoming barriers to community based housing for the chronically mentally ill. *Community Mental Health Journal*, **26**, 330–41.

Wing, J.K. (1962) Institutionalism in mental hospitals. *British Journal of Social and Clinical Psychology*, **1**, 38–51.

Wing, J.K. (1983) Schizophrenia, in *Theory and Practice of Psychiatric Rehabilitation* (eds F.N. Watts and D.H. Bennett), Wiley, Chichester.

Wing, J.K. and Brown G.W. (1970) *Institutionalism and Schizophrenia*, Cambridge University Press, London.

Wing, J.K. and Freudenberg, R.K. (1961) The responses of severely ill chronic schizophrenic patients to social stimulation. *American Journal of Psychiatry*, **118**, 311–22.

Wing, J.K and Morris, B. (1981) *Handbook of Psychiatric Rehabilitation*, Oxford University Press, Oxford.

Wintersteen, R.T. and Rapp, C.A. (1986) The YACP: A dissenting view on an emerging concept. *Psychosocial Rehabilitation Journal*, **9**, 4–13.

Witheridge, T.F. (1989) The assertive community treatment worker: An emerging role and its implications for professional training. *Hospital and Community Psychiatry*, **40**, 620–4.

Wolfensberger, W. and Tullman, S. (1982) A brief outline of the principle of normalisation. *Rehabilitation Psychology*, **27**, 131–45.

Wooff, K. and Goldberg, D.P. (1988) Further observations on the practices of CPNs in Salford: Differences between community psychiatric nurses and mental health social workers. *British Journal of Psychiatry*, **153**, 30–7.

World Federation for Mental Health (1992) Human Rights Bill for Hospitalised Mental Patients. *World Federation for Mental Health Newsletter*, 1992.

Zito Trust (1995) *Learning the Lessons*, Zito Trust, London.

Index